CHAGAS DISEASE

STILL A THREAT TO OUR WORLD?

Tropical Diseases - Etiology, Pathogenesis and Treatments

Additional books in this series can be found on Nova's website under the Series tab.

Additional e-books in this series can be found on Nova's website under the e-book tab.

TROPICAL DISEASES - ETIOLOGY, PATHOGENESIS AND TREATMENTS

CHAGAS DISEASE

STILL A THREAT TO OUR WORLD?

FERNANDA RAMOS GADELHA

AND

EDUARDO DE FIGUEIREDO PELOSO

EDITORS

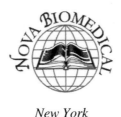

New York

Library of Congress Cataloging-in-Publication Data

ISBN: 978-1-62808-681-2

Library of Congress Control Number: 2013945708

Published by Nova Science Publishers, Inc. † *New York*

To my Mom, Ralf Francisco and special friends that are always with me...
inside my heart

Fernanda

To all my family, especially my mother and father, and all the special
people who live in my heart

Eduardo

Contents

Foreword

In the years that followed the discovery of the disease by Carlos Chagas there was an unfortunate and lasting controversy, since influential local medical groups refused to give the proper credit to the true discoverer of the disease. A newspaper of the time reported a meeting of the National Academy of Medicine, Rio de Janeiro, in November of 1923 (14 years after the original report of the disease!) in which the discussion was no longer centered on the importance of the disease, but rather on who was, in fact, its discoverer. The attempts to deny the accomplishments of Carlos Chagas raised the attention even of a former President of Brazil, Epitácio Pessoa, who had recently left office. He sent a handwritten message to the scientist on the news snippet: "Mediocrity does not forgive talent as darkness does not forgive light. Epitácio Pessoa 9-21-1923" [1]. Due to the importance of its discovery, and also to the relevance of the discoverer for Brazilian science, it never suffices to write about the disease and update the international literature with new knowledge on epidemiology, pathology and clinical aspects of Chagas disease as well as on the molecular mechanisms involved in the ailment. That is the aim of this excellent initiative organized by Fernanda Ramos Gadelha of the University of Campinas (UNICAMP), São Paulo.

The World Health Organization estimates that Chagas disease was responsible for the death, in 2008, of more than 10,000 people from a universe of 10 million who were infected with *Trypanosoma cruzi*. Social and economic conditions such as poverty in Iberoamerican countries, associated on the one hand with political insecurity and, on the other, with the attraction exerted by wealth and social stability in developed countries, has catalyzed the appearance of important migratory currents to the USA, Europe and Japan. As a consequence Chagas disease, which is still a neglected disease restricted to South America and to the South of North America, is being slowly transformed into a new global menace to human health.

In fact, estimates point to 300,000 people infected with the parasite in the USA out of, approximately, 22 to 23 million immigrants from Iberoamerica (numbers of 2005). In Australia, 4% of the 150,000 immigrants who arrived there in 2006 were carriers of the protozoon. Of the 1.7 million immigrants from Iberoamerica admitted into Spain in 2008, 17,500 developed symptoms of the disease [2]. It is possible that the increase in Chagas disease cases in developed countries is due to increasing poverty as a consequence of economic difficulties as well as from the relative inexperience of the health sector in the clinical and serological diagnosis of the disease.

Some authors [3] correlate the expansion of Chagas disease in the USA to the decline of sanitary vigilance, to relatively lower budgets for epidemiological services and to the deepening of social inequality. Accordingly, the disease is particularly prevalent in the Gulf Coast States, such as Louisiana, Mississipi and Alabama, where poverty affects 20% of the population and 2.8 million children live in houses where income is less that US$ 2 per person per day. Furthermore, an increase in infected Triatomines has been found in the USA. From 164 insects (*Triatoma rubida*) collected in domiciles and in the peridomicile in Arizona, 41.5% were infected with *Trypanosoma cruzi* [4].

Successful initiatives to combat parasite transmission are all of epidemiological character. With the guidance of WHO and the efficient collaboration of health ministries, huge programs have been implanted in the last two decades in Brazil, Chile, Uruguay and Argentina to eliminate the insect vector via several systems of treating homes and the environment with insecticides. As a consequence, a dramatic fall in parasite transmission indices by the insect vector has been observed. Obviously, such measures do not solve the problem of already infected people nor do they block transmission by the placenta or by food, when, inadvertently, people ingest juices of sugar cane or açaí, for example, contaminated with crushed insects.

The only drug that remains in the market is Rochagan (Benznidazole), but the manufacturer has foreclosed its production and assigned the license to a Brazilian public laboratory (LAFEPE, Pernambuco). Nevertheless, this medicine although efficient in the acute phase of the disease, is rather toxic and, in spite of the efforts of clinical investigators, is inefficient in the chronic phase. At least consortia, such as Drugs for Neglected Diseases Initiative (DNDi) and the Consortium for Parasitic Drug Development and Institute for One World Health (IoWH), are trying new drugs in pre-clinical trials, such as Posoconazol and Ravuconazol, and K777, an inhibitor of cruzipain.

Hence, research ought to concentrate on the development of efficient drugs that kill the parasite but, preferentially, not the host, and also on vaccines. Besides the fact that several trials to protect experimental animals with isolated antigens were not very successful, for logistic reasons a preventive vaccine has little chances of success. However, the development of a DNA therapeutic vaccine maintains hopes for finding a medicine that would avoid, at least, the appearance of the lesions that determine cardiomyopathy and megaviscera [5].

Basic studies with *Trypanosoma cruzi* performed since the seventies have helped to identify new classes of molecules and biological mechanisms and have been important in depicting the molecular profile of the parasite, important for the rational design of drugs. These studies have brought to the forefront many Iberoamerican groups of investigators who transformed the protozoon into a biological system in an amenable format that has attracted the attention of competent groups from the Northern Hemisphere.

Trypanosoma cruzi is a eukaryote, but its genome may have few introns, if any. The genes are grouped into constitutive expressed operons. The control of gene expression does not occur at the transcription initiation, but rather at that of post-transcriptional mechanisms and mRNA processing occurs by trans-splicing [cf.6]. Moreover, the DNA pre-replication complex is dissimilar to that from higher eukaryotes, resembling that found in Archea [7]. Much work has been invested in trying to understand how the parasite recognizes host-cell receptors and in identifying the downstream signals that are activated upon parasite docking onto the host cell. Currently, investigators are examining the mutual interrelationship between the metabolisms of the intracellular amastigote form and the host-cell. Hopefully, knowledge of the parasite molecular pathways may uncover sites for specific drug targeting.

Despite the fact that a cure for the disease has not, as yet, been achieved, in the past 40 years there has been considerable progress in the understanding of the parasite, the vectors and the pathology of the disease. This book provides up to date information on several aspects of the disease, ranging from historical aspects right up to the targets for therapeutic intervention, touching on recent epidemiological surveys, as well as novelties in clinical and laboratory diagnosis. It will be useful to students and scientists who wish to obtain information on a still neglected disease, but one which is on the brink of becoming a respected and universally feared illness.

Walter Colli
Professor of Biochemistry
University of São Paulo
Brazil

References

[1]   Kropf SP, de Lacerda AL (2009) *In:* Carlos Chagas, Scientist of Brazil, p. 161, Fiocruz ed., Rio de Janeiro, 306 pp.

[2]   Coura JR, Viñas PA. Chagas disease: a new worldwide challenge. *Nature.* 2010; 465: S6-7.

[3]   Hotez PJ. America's Most Distressed Areas and Their Neglected Infections: The United States Gulf Coast and the District of Columbia. *PLoS Negl. Trop. Dis.* 2011; 5 (3) e843.

[4]   Reisenman CE, Lawrence G, Guerestein PG, Gregory T, Dotson E, Hildebrand JG Infection of Kissing Bugs with *Trypanosoma cruzi, Emerg. Infect. Dis.* 2010; 16: 400-5.

[5]   Dumonteil E, Bottazzi ME, Zhan B, Heffernan MJ, Jones K, Valenzuela JG, Kamhawi S, Ortega J, Rosales SPL, Lee BY, Bacon KM, Fleischer B, Slingsby BT, Cravioto MB, Tapia-Conyer R, Hotez PJ. Accelerating the development of a therapeutic vaccine for human Chagas disease: rationale and prospects. *Expert Rev. Vaccines.* 2012; 11:1043–55.

[6]   Serpeloni M, Moraes CB, Muniz JRC, Motta MCM, Ramos ASP, Kessler RL, Inoue AH, DaRocha WD, Yamada-Ogatta SF, Fragoso SP, Goldenberg S, Freitas Jr LH, Ávila AR. An Essential Nuclear Protein in Trypanosomes is a Component of mRNA Transcription/Export Pathway. *PLoS One.* 2011; 6 (6), e20730.

[7]   da Silva MS, da Silveira RCV, Perez AM, Monteiro JP, Calderano SG, da Cunha JP, Elias MC, Cano MIN. Nuclear DNA Replication in Trypanosomatid Protozoa, *In*: DNA Replication and Mutation (Leitner, R.P., ed.), 123-177, Nova Science Publishers, Inc., Hauppauge, New York. 2012.

Acknowledgments

Carlos Chagas and all the researchers whose scientific research gave us the foundation on which we build our own

The financial agencies Fundação de Amparo a Pesquisa do Estado de São Paulo (FAPESP), Conselho Nacional de Desenvolvimento Científico e Tecnológico (CNPq) and (Capes) for grant supports and fellowships.

To God, for all the opportunities, and our families and friends, who encouraged us and supported us during the preparation of this book.

In: Chagas Disease   ISBN: 978-1-62808-681-2
Editors: F. R. Gadelha, E.d.F. Peloso   © 2013 Nova Science Publishers, Inc.

Chapter I

Chagas Disease in Brazil: Historical Aspects[*]

Simone Petraglia Kropf
Graduate Program in the History of Science and Health,
Casa de Oswaldo Cruz, Fundação Oswaldo Cruz, Rio de Janeiro-RJ, Brazil

Abstract

This chapter analyzes the historical process by which American trypanosomiasis, or Chagas disease, described by Carlos Chagas in April 1909, came to be defined and recognized as a scientific fact and public health problem in Brazil. Two periods of the process are addressed. The first covers Chagas' research from 1909 until his death in 1934, when certain pronouncements about the illness gave rise to a heated debate that encompassed the issues of the "backwardness" of the Brazilian interior, the relation between rural endemic diseases and national identity, and the social role of science as a key instrument in Brazilian modernization. In the second half of the 1910s, this debate culminated in the so-called sanitation movement, while in the early 1920s it ignited a fierce controversy over the medical and social import of the disease. The second period focuses on studies led by disciples of Chagas from 1935 to the

---

[*] This chapter is a modified version of the text "Medicina tropical no Brasil: a construção científica e social da doença de Chagas (1909-1962)," published in NASCIMENTO, D.R., CARVALHO, D.M., editors, *Uma história brasileira das doenças* (v. 3) (Belo Horizonte: Argvmentvm, 2010, 257-291). English version by Diane Grosklaus Whitty.

early 1960s. These resulted in new knowledge and in agreement about the clinical and social definition of the disease, eventually gaining it full medical and scientific recognition and its inclusion on the Brazilian State's public health agenda.

Introduction

In April 1909, Carlos Chagas (1878-1934) announced to the scientific world that he had discovered a new tropical disease in the interior of the state of Minas Gerais, in southern Brazil, caused by the protozoan *Trypanosoma cruzi* – likewise described by him, in late 1908 – and transmitted by a hematophagous insect popularly known as the *barbeiro*, or kissing bug, which infested the typical wattle-and-daub homes of the rural poor. The discovery was exulted as a triumph for Brazilian science and, more specifically, for experimental medicine, underpinned by the new theories of microbiology and tropical medicine. Chagas, a researcher at the Oswaldo Cruz Institute (Instituto Oswaldo Cruz, or IOC; also known as Manguinhos Institute), gained great scientific renown in Brazil and abroad and went on to lead a notable public life as director both of the IOC (1917-1934) and of federal health services (1919-1926) [1, 2].

The discovery of Chagas disease played a major role in the institutionalization and legitimization of Brazilian science in the early decades of the twentieth century. The event was promptly recognized as going beyond the scientific accomplishments of a single individual. It represented not only the active involvement and participation of Brazilians in the global movement to institutionalize Mansonian tropical medicine – which was living its golden age – but also reflected the specific social identity then attached to biomedical science as practiced in Brazil at research institutes like the IOC. Chagas' achievement made an original contribution to the era's emerging knowledge about the relation between vectors, parasites, and human diseases and came to symbolize a brand of science that sought to combine knowledge production attuned to the international scientific agenda with a social commitment to identifying and solving Brazil's concrete public health problems. By adding rural endemic diseases to the public agenda as obstacles to the nation's progress, the issue of Chagas disease provided a new framework for looking at Brazil, from a perspective that identified the sound health of the population – especially people living in the rural areas of this agrarian export country – as the basic prerequisite for Brazil's joining the so-called concert of civilized nations, so widely hailed in the early days of the twentieth century [3].

The road to recognizing Chagas disease as both a medical and social issue was, however, not as smooth and straight as traditional accounts of Carlos Chagas' feat would lead us to believe. Following an initial period of great attention from the scientific world and in public life in Brazil, the whole matter of Chagas disease came up against a series of challenges, which in fact revealed the close link between the scientific and political dimensions of the topic [4]. The disease was only to become fully accepted as a medical fact and a national public health issue in the first decades following the death of Carlos Chagas, when his disciples took up the task of ensuring continuity of his research agenda; within Brazil's new historical conjuncture, his followers likewise reasserted the issue of rural endemic diseases as the cornerstone of a scientific and social project, even bringing into its folds social groups outside the specific realms of science [3]. Let us examine the principle milestones of these two periods, marked by continuities and differences yet decisive to the construction of an enduring tradition in Brazilian science and health, with the participation of many generations from a broad spectrum of Brazilian social life, inside the laboratory and out.

Discovery in – and of – Rural Brazil

Carlos Chagas made the discovery that earned him acclaim within the historical context of a modernization project implemented by the newly proclaimed Brazilian Republic, which was swept up in the enthusiasm of "new times" while simultaneously grappling with the challenges of laying the path to the much longed-for "civilization of the tropics." Although this "dream of progress" could boast as its emblem a beautified Rio de Janeiro, then federal capital, which had undergone extensive urban reform evoking Europe's Belle Époque at the dawn of the twentieth century, if the vast territory of Brazil was to be settled and integrated into the nation, this progress would also require infrastructure works in the interior of what was basically a rural country. It was during one of these vital modernization projects – the extension of the Central do Brasil railway from Rio de Janeiro to northern Brazil – that Carlos Chagas was dispatched to the north of Minas Gerais, in June 1907, to combat a malaria epidemic that had halted construction of the track between Corinto and Pirapora.

Born on a farm in the small city of Oliveira, Minas Gerais, Carlos Chagas had graduated from the Rio de Janeiro School of Medicine in 1903. At the newly created Manguinhos Institute, with Oswaldo Cruz serving as his advisor, Chagas had chosen to write his medical thesis on malaria, then on the order of the day in Mansonian tropical medicine. While at medical school, he had been introduced to the topic by Francisco Fajardo, a pioneer of microbiology and tropical medicine in Brazil.

By the time he made the trip to Minas, Chagas had already led two anti-malaria campaigns, one in Itatinga, São Paulo, and the other in Xerém, located in the Baixada Fluminense area of the state of Rio de Janeiro, both under assignment by Oswaldo Cruz, then director general of public health as well as director of the Manguinhos Institute. After Chagas set up temporary office in 1907 in the small settlement of São Gonçalo das Tabocas (renamed Lassance in February 1908), he combined his anti-malaria endeavors with research into the local fauna, spurred by his interest in protozoology and entomology, which were key areas on the research agenda at the IOC, where he would become an assistant researcher in March 1908.

That year, through engineer Cornélio Cantarino Motta, Chagas made acquaintance with the barbeiro insects that infested the region's mud-walled houses. Well aware of the role that hematophagous insects play in the transmission of parasitic diseases, Chagas examined some specimens of these kissing bugs and identified in their intestines a flagellated protozoan in the form of a trypanosome. Not long before, he had described *Trypanosoma minasense*, found in sagui monkeys from the region. Trypanosomes were then drawing the attention of researchers in the field of European tropical medicine, who were studying and fighting African trypanosomiasis. Chagas kept abreast of this research primarily through exchanges between Manguinhos researchers and German protozoologists [3, 5].

To better investigate the nature of the parasite found in the barbeiros, Chagas sent specimens to Oswaldo Cruz so he could conduct experiments with the saguis raised at the Manguinhos laboratories. When Chagas learned that one of the monkeys had contracted the infection from the flagellate, he returned to Rio and concluded that this was a new species of trypanosome, which he named *Trypanosoma cruzi* in honor of his mentor Oswaldo Cruz. Convinced that *T. cruzi* could be pathogenic to humans, he went back to Lassance and performed systematic tests on residents there. On April 14, 1909, he observed the parasite in the blood of a feverish two-year-old girl named Berenice. He announced the first case of a new human trypanosomiasis in a preliminary note published in *Brazil-Medico* [6]. At the suggestion of Miguel

Couto, professor at the Rio de Janeiro School of Medicine and a major influence on Chagas during his academic training, the disease was termed "moléstia de Chagas," or "Chagas disease."

This threefold discovery was soon celebrated as a great triumph for Brazilian science, and many considered it a unique event in the history of medicine, since a single researcher had described a new disease, its transmitter, and its causative agent, all in a brief period of time. Chagas went on to become a member of the top medical and scientific associations in Brazil and abroad. In 1910, he was made a fellow of Brazil's prestigious National Academy of Medicine (Academia Nacional de Medicina, or ANM). In 1912, he won the Schaudinn Prize in protozoology, awarded by the Hamburg Institute for Maritime and Tropical Diseases, and the following year he received his first nomination for a Nobel Prize in medicine (his second came in 1921).

Research into the new disease became the flagship of Oswaldo Cruz's project to build the IOC into a renowned center for research in experimental medicine (especially tropical medicine) that would address the country's public health issues [7, 8].[1] Chagas enjoyed the collaboration of a number of researchers, who provided essential contributions to investigations of various aspects of the new illness. Gaspar Vianna studied the parasite's characteristics – such as its reproduction within tissues – and the pathogeny of the disease; Arthur Neiva described different species of triatomines and their distribution across Brazil; Ezequiel Dias addressed hematological aspects of infection with *T. cruzi*; Carlos Bastos de Magarinos Torres concentrated on the pathology of the disease; Astrogildo Machado tested several medications in the quest for a therapeutic resource and, working with Cesar Guerreiro, developed the first serological method for diagnosing *T. cruzi* infection, known as the Machado-Guerreiro reaction; and, lastly, Eurico Villela devoted himself to clinical study of the disease, especially its cardiac form.

From his earliest publications, Chagas affirmed that the new trypanosomiasis did permanent damage to the physical and mental development of the rural folk living in the mud-walled, thatched-roof huts known as *cafuas*, which abounded with barbeiros. This endemic disease, he argued, presented a serious menace to national progress, and government

---

[1] The Federal Serum Therapy Institute (Instituto Soroterápico Federal), also known as Manguinhos Institute, was inaugurated in 1900 to manufacture bubonic plague serum and vaccine for use in the fight against an epidemic that was threatening to strike Rio de Janeiro. In 1908, it was renamed the Oswaldo Cruz Institute after its director. Today it is one of the scientific units of the Oswaldo Cruz Foundation.

authorities should combat it decisively. The new tropical malady identified in the hinterlands of Minas Gerais thus acquired an emblematic significance as the "disease of Brazil" – a manifestation of national identity not just in a geographic sense but in numerous other ways. It became the symbol of an "ailing country," where endemic diseases jeopardized the dream of attaining "civilization" by compromising the productivity of rural laborers; furthermore, it symbolized the science that had "discovered" this unknown Brazil and would lead its incorporation into the march of national progress. It was a case that exemplified how Brazilian scientists appropriated concepts and theories from European tropical medicine and then used these to produce original contributions to knowledge in the field, with specific applications to Brazilian reality [3].

Encountering the Disease of the Hinterlands

On October 26, 1910, the day he became a fellow of the National Academy of Medicine, Chagas presented the first clinical characterization of the disease. According to the Brazilian scientist, the main symptoms of the acute phase were fever; enlarged liver, spleen, and lymph nodes; and facial swelling (mixedema), the latter considered a sign of a compromised thyroid. Chagas divided this phase into two forms: cases entailing serious brain disorders (generally involving children under the age of one, who rarely survived) and more common cases, devoid of any such manifestations, which evolved to the chronic stage within a month [9].

The chronic phase, into which most cases allegedly fell, was defined as encompassing endocrinological, cardiac, and neurological disturbances. Chagas believed that the most characteristic clinical sign in the first group was hypertrophy of the thyroid (goiter). Convinced that *T. cruzi* damaged this gland, Chagas formulated the hypothesis that in Minas Gerais and other regions of *T. cruzi* infection, endemic goiter was not the same as in Europe but was instead a clinical manifestation of trypanosomiasis. Chagas further believed that chronic infection included a "nervous form" as well, triggered by the parasite's location in the central nervous system and the cause of motor dysfunctions, speech problems, and cognitive issues, especially in children. According to Chagas, *T. cruzi* also damaged the myocardium, provoking alterations in cardiac rhythm. The "cardiac form" presented in young adults in the prime of their productive lives. The prognosis was usually serious, leading to heart failure and in some cases sudden death [9]. It was Oswaldo Cruz himself who announced the discovery of Chagas disease and associated research to the medical community, heralding it as a major victory for Brazilian science. Cruz took his young disciple's accomplishment as a unique opportunity to strengthen the IOC's project as an institute committed to the interests of Brazilian society and to advancing knowledge in prominent areas of international science [7,8]. In addition to personally announcing Chagas' discovery before the ANM, Oswaldo Cruz proposed that the Academy send a commission comprising Miguel Pereira, Miguel Couto, Antonio Austregésilo, Juliano Moreira, and Antonio Fernandes Figueira to Lassance in 1910 to witness and validate Chagas' research.

Bearing a stamp of approval from the luminaries of Brazilian medicine, Chagas' ideas started to circulate and to lend form to an issue that was both medical and social. As of 1910, Chagas began to systematically iterate that when Brazilian science and society had become aware of this new disease entity, they had encountered an illness that revealed structural facets of Brazilian reality and its problems. In his first conference before the ANM, in October 1910, Chagas stated that the disease was a "terrible scourge over a vast area of the country, where it renders countless people unfit for life's activities and produces successive generations of inferior men, of useless individuals, fatally damned to chronic morbidity, displaying such a coefficient of inferiority that they have become worthless to the progressive evolution of our Fatherland" [9]. His words were punctuated by a very persuasive strategy. The night of Chagas' first conference, the Academy inaugurated its electric lighting as yet another symbol of the progress being celebrated in the newly reformed capital of the Belle Époque. But the power source was used to project cinematographic images of the ill in Lassance, materializing the faces of a Brazil that was the antithesis of so-called civilization. Laboratory equipment was also used to convince the eminent audience, with microscopes made available to anyone wishing to observe the new parasite. The press then reported on this "show," transmitting Chagas' thoughts to an even larger audience [3].

Characterized as the illness of the hinterlands, Chagas disease translated the notion of "tropical disease" as a "national disease." If, as David Arnold [10] has submitted, European contact with the tropics – as a physical, conceptual, cultural, and political space – constituted an experience of Otherness, the characterization of trypanosomiasis also revealed an Other. Chagas' formulations combined knowledge production, social indictment, and political grievance: "Will it be possible, within public hygiene, to find efficacious ways of attenuating this affliction? We believe so, if this problem – most surely a problem of the State and of humanity – becomes the concern of a scientifically well-advised statesman" [9]. During the 1910 debate over Chagas disease, there emerged the rallying cries which years later would galvanize the medical and hygienist movement that wanted to see the "sanitizing" of the hinterlands and related reforms to Brazil's federal public health services.

In 1911, at a second ANM conference, this time before Brazilian President Hermes da Fonseca, Chagas painted an even stronger bond between the medical-scientific elements of this disease and the features that shaped it as a social issue. The IOC researcher stated that trypanosomiasis was not only prejudicial to progress in already populated areas of the hinterlands but also hampered further territorial settlement. Where population hubs sprang up, accompanying the expansion of the railroad (like Lassance), primitive housing constructions vulnerable to infestation by kissing bugs became foci for the disease. The barbeiro's notable capacity to transmit *T. cruzi*, its long lifespan, its resistance to lengthy periods of fasting, and the ease with which it could be transported in baggage made the bug a powerful enemy that could "settle" many regions of the country, keeping pace with economic advances and internal migration. Citing the Europeans who were endeavoring to combat African trypanosomiasis and other tropical diseases in the defense of colonialist interests, Chagas drove home the idea that studies of tropical medicine in Brazil should be for the benefit of the nation: "We must safeguard the future of a great people" [11].

At the same time that Brazil was learning about studies of the new disease, the topic was garnering attention on the international stage, especially in the realm of European tropical medicine. In addition to articles in foreign journals, trypanosomiasis was also a highlighted theme at the Brazilian pavilion of the International Exposition on Hygiene and Demography in Dresden, Germany, in 1911.

During the first years that knowledge was being produced about the disease, the relation between its scientific and its political-social dimensions was expressed primarily in writings and statements by Chagas, featured in arenas of medical science like laboratories, the specialized literature, congresses, and medical associations. But as of 1916, new audiences began engaging in the process, and the topic entered the broader political debate about the nation.

Between Doubts and Triumphs:
The Disease of Brazil and
the Sanitation Movement

In 1915, research conducted in Argentina under the leadership of Austrian microbiologist Rudolf Kraus cast doubts on Chagas' formulations about the chronic forms of trypanosomiasis, especially the correlation with endemic goiter. Although infected barbeiros and goiter sufferers were found in Argentina, researchers there were bothered by the fact that not a single human case of the disease had been diagnosed in the country in parasitological terms [12, 13].[2] They argued that the thyroidal and neurological manifestations attributed to the chronic phase of American trypanosomiasis in fact represented the endemic goiter and cretinism found in Europe – in other words, they were distinct yet overlapping endemic illnesses. For them, trypanosomiasis was essentially an acute disease, limited to the locations where it had been studied in Brazil. They held that the Argentinean climate might possibly attenuate the virulence of *T. cruzi*, accounting for the absence of cases in that country.[3]

In September 1916, Chagas contested these allegations at a medical congress in Buenos Aires. He stated that even if he should come to revise some of his ideas, he did not feel his overall concept of the disease – which, he pointed out, was restricted neither to acute cases nor to Brazil – was at risk. Nevertheless, even while reiterating his convictions, he commenced a significant process of reformulation of the clinical profile of trypanosomiasis, which downplayed the primacy of thyroidal signs and underscored the importance of cardiac elements. In his proposed new classification for the chronic forms, he presented the parasitic etiology of endemic goiter as a "related problem," open to review [15].

In October, at a ceremony at the Rio de Janeiro School of Medicine, physician and Professor Miguel Pereira made the speech that would become famous as the point of origin of the sanitation movement. This campaign, which was formalized in 1918 with the creation of the Pro-Sanitation League of Brazil, brought physicians, scientists, intellectuals, and politicians together around the idea that Brazilian backwardness was not a result of its tropical

---

[2] One of the points that elicited questions was the fact that the method Chagas used to demonstrate the presence of the parasite in chronic cases had been refuted in 1913.

[3] The first record of acute cases of the disease in Argentina dates to 1924 [14].

climate or of the racial makeup of its people but of the appalling public health conditions prevalent in its vast interior [16]. World War I formed a backdrop for an environment of fervent nationalism, and topics like the racial question, immigration, and military recruitment intersected within attempts to identify the country's ills as well as opportunities for its "regeneration". Pereira was upset by those who exhorted Brazilians to engage in the defense of civic and patriotic values without paying any heed to rural Brazil's real living and health conditions. He summed up his indignation with a metaphor that would become legendary: "Brazil is still an enormous hospital" [17]. This indictment of Brazil as an enormous hospital was greatly informed by the significance accorded to Chagas disease. The relation was recognized by Belisário Penna himself, chief leader of the sanitary movement, who stated: "Chagas' noteworthy discovery. . .was the drop that pushed the great master's chalice of indignation to overflowing and instilled in him the courage to articulate [this indignation] through his renowned phrase, for it is painfully and profoundly true" [18].[4]

The fact that American trypanosomiasis and Carlos Chagas were on center stage in the political realm was a badge of recognition and a source of legitimacy, but it also left the door open to more criticisms and tension. As the "disease of Brazil" spurred sanitarians on, it became the center of a heated controversy, where the scientific dimension was tightly associated with the political content of the debate.

National Calamity or "Sickness of Lassance"? The Disease of Brazil in Question

In 1919, some Brazilian researchers took up the arguments presented in Argentina. They questioned the clinical definition of American trypanosomiasis and especially its social importance. Within the National Academy of Medicine, the controversy grew more heated in late 1922 and 1923. Led by Julio Afrânio Peixoto (1876-1947), a renowned man of letters

---

[4] In October 1919, Chagas took over as head of Brazil's federal public health services. In response to grievances put forward by the sanitation movement, the services were re-organized, which included the January 1920 creation of the National Department of Public Health (Departamento Nacional de Saúde Pública, or DNSP) [19]. Chagas served as head of the DNSP (1920-1926) while also director of the IOC (1917-1934).

who held the chair in hygiene at the University of Rio de Janeiro's School of Medicine, Chagas' critics asserted that this was a rare disease restricted to the region of Lassance and not a national scourge. According to them, the notion of a "diseased Brazil" disseminated by Chagas and followers of the rural sanitation movement was exaggerated and pessimistic and, furthermore, discredited Brazil and scared off immigrants and foreign capital.

They also questioned the pathogenicity of *Trypanosoma cruzi* and the authorship of its discovery, which, some argued, fell not to Chagas but to Oswaldo Cruz, since the latter had conducted the experiments that made it possible to identify the new parasite. There was much press coverage of the clash, which involved not just scientific matters but political ones as well, tied to the era's passionate nationalist debate. This discord was further fed by personal rivalries and conflicts with Chagas, involving his work as director of both the Oswaldo Cruz Institute and the National Department of Public Health.

In its official affidavit, the National Academy of Medicine endorsed Chagas' merits and his authorship of the discovery of *T. cruzi*. However, it took no stance when it came to the disease's clinical definition or geographical range, claiming it was unable to do so. At a crowded session on December 6, Chagas presented a conference at the Academy that finalized the discussions. He indicated what he considered the "indisputable signs" [20] of the clinical definition of trypanosomiasis, like cardiac aspects, while harshly criticizing Peixoto and his spokesmen for their "false nationalism" in trying to "divert the State's efforts away from one of the matters of utmost urgency to our commitment as Brazilians" [20].[5]

This controversy constituted a watershed in Chagas' biography and in the trajectory of trypanosomiasis. Although Chagas himself recognized his conflict with Kraus as essentially scientific in spirit, the idea began to hold sway – especially after his death – that Chagas had come up against "detractors." For Carlos Chagas Filho [1], the disputes were motivated not only by jealousy over the approbation his father enjoyed but also by designs on the posts of director of Manguinhos and of the National Department of Public Health. Benchimol and Teixeira [8] have pointed out that the problems Chagas faced as head of the IOC and DNSP lay at the crux of these clashes. Coutinho, Freire Jr. and Dias [21] argue that the conflicts explain why Chagas did not receive the Nobel Prize in medicine for which he was nominated in 1921. Another point often reiterated is that the episode within the ANM

---

[5] For a thoroughgoing analysis of this discussion in the ANM, see [3, 4].

relegated the disease to a period of discredit or oblivion, compromising the continuity of studies on the topic [1, 22].

According to Stepan [23], the conflict at the ANM had to do with the debate about tropical medicine in Brazil and its implications for national identity. Peixoto's reactions to the representation of Brazil as an enormous hospital signaled his negation of the idea of a kind of medicine specific to the tropics. For him, the notion of tropical diseases was unacceptable as it amounted to a rehashing of longstanding European stereotypes and biases about the tropics as places adverse to civilization, grounded in a climatic determinism incompatible with the "redemptive" perspectives of hygiene.

The controversy surrounding American trypanosomiasis presented components of a scientific nature – that is, very real doubts about the clinical and epidemiological characterization of the disease at that time – and of a political nature as well. It went beyond rivalries with Chagas and beyond the matter of the criticisms to which he was subjected as a public figure, embodying a collision between two positions within the era's nationalist debate: the defense versus the negation of the diagnosis of Brazil as an "enormous hospital," with both positions sharing the view that Chagas disease was the emblem of this vision of the nation [3,4].

Back to Argentina and to the Hinterlands of Minas: Studies on the Disease after Carlos Chagas

Although Chagas forged ahead with his studies, delving deeper into cardiac aspects of the disease, these controversies bred a climate of doubt and uncertainty that would only be settled after his death, which took place in November 1934. A first crucial step in this process was the research conducted by the Misión de Estudios de Patología Regional Argentina (Mepra), created in 1926 and led by physician Salvador Mazza. One of the milestones of these studies was Cecílio Romaña's 1935 description of a clinical sign that afforded an easy and immediate diagnosis of acute cases. This was unilateral schizotrypanosic conjunctivitis, a swelling of the eyelids that signals the infection's portal of entry, where an inflammatory reaction occurs in response to the penetration of *T. cruzi* in the conjunctiva, through the barbeiro's contaminated feces. The announcement of "Romaña's sign" led to the diagnosis of hundreds of cases in Argentina [14] and elsewhere within a few years, greatly encouraging those in Brazil who wanted to further advance Carlos Chagas' research [3].

Among these was Chagas' eldest son, Evandro Chagas, who was conducting research on the cardiac form of the disease and who in 1937 established the Service for Studies on Major Endemic Diseases (Serviço de Estudos de Grandes Endemias, or SEGE) at the IOC. Inspired on his father's sanitation ideals, the project was meant to establish regional institutes to study the main diseases of rural Brazil and to support sanitary services in the fight against these illnesses, in cooperation with state governments. In 1939, in conjunction with researchers from the Ezequiel Dias Biological Institute (Instituto Biológico Ezequiel Dias, or IBED, the former branch of the IOC in Belo Horizonte, capital of Minas Gerais state), SEGE defined a research plan for studying Chagas disease and began looking for new cases, using the strategy of making local physicians aware of Romaña's sign. In 1940, an important focus of the disease was discovered in the small western Minas town of Bambuí, and Amilcar Vianna Martins, of the IBED, was assigned to lead its study [24]. After Evandro Chagas passed away in 1940, the direction of SEGE fell to his brother, Carlos Chagas Filho, until 1942, when the service was absorbed by the Division of Studies on Endemic Diseases (Divisão de Estudos de Endemias), created in the early days of Henrique Aragão's term as IOC director.

The World War II context was particularly favorable to Aragão's project to move forward with Manguinhos' research agenda on rural endemic diseases. Around the world, a mood of optimism was being kindled about new preventive and therapeutic resources, like DDT and penicillin, then developed to fight the infectious diseases that were a constant threat to soldiers on the front. Aragão was confident in these new resources; furthermore, the institutional circumstances at Manguinhos were favorable because of growing demand by the Ministry of Education and Health, so he established research posts around the country where rural endemic diseases could be studied and combated, like yaws, schistosomiasis, and Chagas disease. Late 1943 saw creation of the Center for Studies and Prophylaxis on Chagas Disease (Centro de Estudos e Profilaxia da Moléstia de Chagas, or CEPMC), an IOC post in the city of Bambuí, Minas Gerais, whose direction was entrusted to Emmanuel Dias (1908-1962), disciple and godchild of Carlos Chagas; the post would prove decisive to securing scientific and social recognition of trypanosomiasis [3].

In the post-1930 national context, the topic of rural endemic diseases took on new meaning, which was to the advantage of continued studies on Chagas disease at Manguinhos in the decades following Carlos Chagas' death. While Getúlio Vargas' modernization project prioritized the urban industrial world, rural development was vital to ensuring supplies for a national consumer market that would be capable of sustaining the new economic model. In political and ideological terms, the government cast labor as the primary value in the construction of a "new nation," thus providing support for projects intended to guarantee the existence of healthy, strong, productive workers in the city and country [25].

Research by the Oswaldo Cruz Institute In Bambuí

One of the CEPMC's prime goals was to create the technical conditions for an offensive against Chagas disease via a systematic attack on its vectors. In 1944, when DDT was reaping resounding success in the fight against epidemic typhus and malaria among World War II troops, Dias set about testing it on barbeiros, with great expectations. In 1945, however, scientists concluded that it was not effective against the transmitters of Chagas disease. Improved housing was another preventive measure tested by the CEPMC. Dias conducted trials in the search for a simple plastering technique that would keep barbeiros from infesting walls; he implemented experimental construction of "hygienic houses" in Bambuí [26]. In 1948, with the collaboration of Minas Gerais physician José Pellegrino, he tested an insecticide that in laboratory trials proved to have a suitable residual power against barbeiros, making it viable for use in a campaign [27]. Nearly forty years after discovery of the disease, scientists had a concrete weapon against American trypanosomiasis: hexachlorocyclohexane (HCH).

Another aim of the Bambuí post was clinical study of the disease, especially its chronic phase, into which most cases evolved; moreover, the bulk of the doubts about Chagas' formulations also pertained to this phase. During the chronic phase, diagnosis is not possible through direct observation of the blood since the parasite disappears from the bloodstream, and other methods then available did not always yield accurate results (for further information, see chapter 5). It was essential to define criteria for clinical diagnosis that would point the way to sound laboratory tests, like serological exams. The decision was made to invest in researching the cardiac form, which was where greatest consensus lay about the clinical profile outlined by Chagas, even though further clarifications were considered necessary [28].

The collaboration of cardiologist Francisco Laranja – who had vast experience in the use of modern electrocardiography techniques – was vital to the definitive recognition of the cardiac form of Chagas disease [29]. Availing themselves of Laranja's clinical expertise, CEPMC scientists characterized the typical electrocardiographic profile for chronic chagasic cardiopathy and adopted other strategies to reinforce arguments about its clinical presentation. They conducted surveys among random populations, obtaining electrocardiographic results that indicated that among chronic cases which had been serologically confirmed a significant proportion of patients presented the cardiac form. In addition, they experimentally reproduced chronic cardiopathy in dogs inoculated with *T. cruzi* and obtained electrocardiographic, radiological, and clinical characteristics similar to those shown by humans.

In 1948 the scientists concluded: "Our experience acquired in recent years in Bambuí, where we have followed numerous cases, has convinced us that chronic schizotrypanosis finds its clinical expression essentially in a cardiopathy with well-defined anatomopathological, clinical, radiological, and electrocardiographic characters, rendering individualization certain" [30]. The work on chagasic cardiopathy done by scientists at the CEPMC gained international recognition when it was published in the prestigious U.S. medical journal *Circulation* [31].

Besides its research, the CEPMC took up a rather political task, disseminating the topic of Chagas disease and seeking to draw the attention of other social groups. Their prime target was physicians from the interior. Dias published articles in Brazil's chief medical journals, where he provided general information on the disease and also urged doctors to stand alongside scientists as their allies. A response was not long in coming, and Chagas disease soon became a strong element of professional identity for these "clinical doctors from Central Brazil", above all in the 1950s [3, 32].

In the papers that Dias published during the course of the 1940s – directed not only towards physicians but also the public at large, and from a gamut of social sectors, especially in rural areas, like educators, politicians, and public health figures – he argued that the disease was a serious roadblock to the nation's development because, as a cardiac illness, it compromised the productive capacity of rural workers. On the one hand, the chances of diagnosing new cases were enhanced by spreading the idea that the population and rural physicians should perceive sensations of cardiac disturbances as possible signs of the disease. On the other, this also infused the results of the research with a concrete social meaning that was associated with a central dimension of people's lives, thus redoubling its persuasive power. So propagating the idea that Chagas disease was important because it was a heart disease was fundamental to the process of certifying the knowledge which defined chronic chagasic cardiopathy as an essential dimension of the disease [3].

Backed by this new knowledge – about the disease's clinical profile, diagnostic criteria, epidemiological evaluation, and preventive techniques – and by the largest number of case records on Chagas disease ever compiled in one region of the country (about 600 cases in 1948), Dias began pressuring the government to take immediate steps to combat the sickness. In May 1950, Brazil's first preventive campaign against Chagas disease was inaugurated in the city of Uberaba, in the Minas Gerais Triangle, a region that encapsulated expectations about state economic recovery, consonant with the agenda of Milton Campos, then governor. Under the guidance of the CEPMC, the Ministry of Education and Health's National Malaria Service (Serviço Nacional de Malária/Ministério da Educação e Saúde) applied the HCH insecticide in municipalities in western Minas and northern São Paulo, in cooperation with the Minas Gerais State Department of Health (Secretaria de Saúde do Estado de Minas Gerais) [3].

From the Far Corners of Minas Gerais to Brazil and the Rest of the Americas

The 1950 campaign made Chagas disease a major topic in medical, scientific, and public health forums in Brazil and abroad, focusing attention on the knowledge produced in Bambuí and earning it scientific legitimacy while also drawing the interest of new research groups. At the same time, this field of research began to be institutionalized at Brazilian universities, especially the schools of medicine established in regions where the disease was endemic, like Ribeirão Preto (state of São Paulo), the Minas Gerais Triangle, and Goiânia (state of Goiás). Another major milestone in the process of institutionalization was the First International Congress on Chagas Disease, held in Rio de Janeiro in 1959.

Throughout the 1950s, Dias devoted himself to political mobilization efforts to extend the campaign launched in Uberaba into other regions of the country. In addition, by fostering heavy exchange between scientists and governments in various Latin American nations, he endeavored to convince the Pan American Sanitary Bureau to coordinate a plan to combat the disease across the continent. In 1960, the World Health Organization (WHO) sponsored an expert meeting in Washington to draft guidelines for combating and researching the disease [33].

Dias' efforts in the 1950s to broaden scientific interest in the disease and to institutionalize it as an object of national and international public health policies bore a direct link to the post-war context, where the topic of health found new force in a world that was rebuilding itself, heartened by the "dream of development" [34]. Confidence was restored in new technological tools for attaining the long-sought victory over tropical diseases, which were a matter not only of economic importance, as a way of boosting productivity in the so-called Third World, but of political importance as well, as a way of averting the spread of communist ideology in the region. The 1948 creation of the WHO afforded new institutional and symbolic support for projects intended to break what was then defined as the "vicious cycle of disease and poverty" [35].

In the 1960s and 1970s, the process of institutionalization of Chagas disease in the fields of science and public health continued its advance. When molecular biology and genetic engineering injected new energy into the biological sciences in the 1960s and 1970s, the topic began attracting much interest in the halls of basic research. During this period, the key markers of the institutionalization of a Brazilian research community dedicated to Chagas disease were, first of all, the Integrated Program on Endemic Diseases (Programa Integrado de Doenças Endêmicas, or PIDE), established within the National Council for Scientific and Technological Development (Conselho Nacional de Desenvolvimento Científico e Tecnológico, or CNPq) in 1973 and managed by scientists enjoying broad autonomy through the mid-1980s, and, secondly, the Annual Reunions on Basic Research and Annual Reunions on Applied Research on Chagas disease, introduced respectively in 1974 and 1984. Another major marker was the 1975 creation of the WHO's Tropical Diseases Research (TDR) program, where Chagas disease has always been a component.

In 1975, Brazil's Ministry of Health sponsored the first nationwide survey to chart the prevalence of trypanosomiasis, and in the 1980s disease control was expanded to cover the entire country. In 1991, Southern Cone governments signed a joint agreement to interrupt transmission of the vector in the region. In 2006, the WHO granted Brazil a certificate for having interrupted the transmission of the disease by its main vector species, *Triatoma infestans*.

Final Considerations

The road to constructing the "disease of Brazil" and winning scientific and social legitimacy followed a long course. Working under diverse historical circumstances, scientists mobilized a range of groups, institutional spaces, and spheres of social life in shaping the image of a new tropical disease that had been discovered by a scientist from the tropics and that was gradually defined and recognized in terms of meanings and conditions specific to Brazilian science and society. Combining European theories on germs, vectors, and "warm climate" diseases with issues and challenges particular to a nation that wished to be "civilized" and to the science that wanted to lead it, the path from the discovery of a new parasite in the blood of a young girl in the hinterlands and the configuration of a "disease endemic to the American continent" was anything but smooth; to the contrary, it was a process disrupted by clashes and controversies.

But what imbued this centenary research tradition with its overriding meaning was the twofold objective that had characterized the science of Chagas disease since 1909: the production of original knowledge in line with the international agenda, and the identification of concrete initiatives and methods for addressing Brazil's social ills. In other words, this was a science focused on Brazilian health, a science that uncovered Brazilian problems and indicated ways to combat them.

In the twenty-first century, the topic of neglected diseases, or of diseases of poverty, has revived the challenge of discovering how medicine can or must promote health in the collective sense as a crucial dimension of citizenship, or as "a right of all and the duty of the State," to quote the Brazilian Constitution of 1988, composed in an atmosphere of redemocratization. In the early decades of the twentieth century, physicians like Carlos Chagas shared a vision of the social dimensions of medicine which laid down foundations that helped orient our current directions [36]. The legacy of the past is less about victories and more about questions, which should be brought into the twenty-first century. How can Brazilian medicine play an active role in the global scientific community while rendering appropriate services and devising public policy that responds to the health needs of the Brazilian people, especially the needs of those groups for whom sickness and poverty are two sides of the same coin? This was Chagas' challenge, and today it remains the challenge for those who believe that studying the diseases of Brazil is a reference point for identity and for social action.

References

[1]   Chagas FC. Meu Pai. *Rio de Janeiro: COC/Fiocruz*; 1993.

[2]   Kropf SP, Lacerda AL. Carlos Chagas, scientist of Brasil. Rio de Janeiro: *Editora Fiocruz*; 2009.

[3]   Kropf SP. Doença de Chagas, doença do Brasil: ciência, saúde e nação (1909-1962). Rio de Janeiro: *Editora Fiocruz;* 2009.

[4]   Kropf SP. Carlos Chagas and the debates and controversies surrounding the 'disease of Brazil' (1909-1923). História, Ciências, Saúde – Manguinhos (on-line). 2009, 16 (suplemento). Available from: *http://www.scielo.br/scielo.php?script=sci_arttext&pid=S0104-59702009000500010&lng=en&nrm=iso&tlng=en*

[5]   Kropf SP, SÁ MR. The discovery of *Trypanosoma cruzi* and Chagas disease (1908-1909): tropical medicine in Brazil. História, Ciências, Saúde – Manguinhos. 2009, 16 (supl. 1), 13-34. Available from: http://www.scielo.br/pdf/hcsm/v16s1/02.pdf

[6]   Chagas C. "Nova especie mórbida do homem, produzida por um *Trypanozoma (Trypanozoma cruzi)*: Nota prévia," *Brazil-Medico*, 1909, 23 (16), 161.

[7]   Stepan NL. *Beginnings of Brazilian science. Oswaldo Cruz, medical research and policy, 1890-1920.* New York: Science History Publications, 1976.

[8]   Benchimol JL, Teixeira LA. Cobras, Lagartos & Outros Bichos: uma história comparada dos institutos Oswaldo Cruz e Butantan. *Rio de Janeiro: Editora UFRJ*; 1993.

[9]   Chagas C. Nova entidade morbida do homem. *Brazil-Medico*, 1910, 24(43, 44, 45): 423-428, 433-437, 443-447.

[10]   Arnold D. *Warm Climates and Western Medicine: the emergence of Tropical Medicine, 1500-1900.* Amsterdam, Atlanta: Rodopi; 1996.

[11]   Chagas C. Molestia de Carlos Chagas: Conferencia realizada em 7 de agosto na Academia Nacional de Medicina. *Brazil-Médico*, 1911, 25(34, 35, 36, 37), 340-343, 353-355, 361-364, 373-375.

[12] Kraus R, Maggio C, Rosenbusch F. Bocio, cretinismo y enfermedad de Chagas. 1ª. Comunicación. *La Prensa Medica Argentina*, 1915, 2(1), 2-5.

[13] Kraus R, Rosenbusch F. Bocio, cretinismo y enfermedad de Chagas. 2ª. Comunicación. *La Prensa Medica Argentina*, 1916, 3(17), 177-180.

[14] Zabala JP. Historia de la enfermedad de Chagas en Argentina: evolución conceptual, institucional y política. *História, Ciências, Saúde – Manguinhos*, 2009, 16 (supl. 1): 57-74.

[15] Chagas C. Processos patojenicos da tripanozomiase americana. *Mem Inst Oswaldo Cruz.* 1916; 8: 5-35.

[16] Lima NT, Hochman G. Condenado pela raça, absolvido pela medicina: o Brasil descoberto pelo movimento sanitarista da Primeira República. In: Maio M, Santos RV, editors, Raça, Ciência e Sociedade. *Rio de Janeiro: Editora Fiocruz, Centro Cultural Banco do Brasil;* 1996.

[17] Jornal do Commercio. A manifestação dos acadêmicos ao professor Aloysio de Castro. *Jornal do Commercio*, 11 oct. 1916, Rio de Janeiro, p. 4.

[18] A noite. O Brasil, um vasto hospital. Em torno da moléstia de Chagas. O que nos diz uma autoridade científica, *A Noite, Rio de Janeiro*, 20 aug. 1920.

[19] Hochman G. A Era do Saneamento: as bases da política de Saúde Pública no Brasil. *1st edition. São Paulo: Hucitec, Anpocs*; 1998.

[20] Academia Nacional de Medicina. Sessão de 6 de dezembro de 1923. *Boletim da Academia Nacional de Medicina*, 1923, 785-814.

[21] Coutinho M, Freire JRO, Dias JCP. The Nobel Enigma: Chagas' nominations for the Nobel Prize. *Mem Inst Oswaldo Cruz.* 1999; 94: 123-29.

[22] Coutinho M. Ninety years of Chagas disease: a success story at the periphery. *Social Studies of Science.* 1999; 29: 519-49.

[23] Stepan NL. Appearances and Disappearances. In: *Picturing Tropical Nature.* London: Reaktion Books; 2001.

[24] Martins AV, Versiani V, Tupinambá A. Sobre 25 casos agudos de molestia de Chagas observados em Minas Gerais. *Mem Inst Ezequiel Dias.* 1939-1940, 3/4, 5-51.

[25] Gomes AMC. *A Invenção do Trabalhismo.* Rio de Janeiro, São Paulo: Iuperj, Vértice; 1988.

[26] Dias E. Um Ensaio de Profilaxia de Moléstia de Chagas. *Rio de Janeiro: Imprensa Nacional;* 1945.

[27] Dias E, Pellegrino J. Alguns ensaios com o gammexane no combate aos transmissores da doença de Chagas. *Brasil-Medico.* 1948; 62(18-20), 185-91.

[28] Yorke W. Chagas' disease. A critical review. *Tropical Diseases Bulletin.* 1937; 34: 275-300.

[29] Laranja F. O olhar da cardiologia: Francisco Laranja e as pesquisas sobre a doença de Chagas. Entrevista concedida a Goldschmidt, R.; Benchimol, J. & Chor Maio, M. Apresentação: Hamilton, W. *História, Ciências, Saúde – Manguinhos.* 2009; 16: 95-114.

[30] Laranja F, Dias E, Nóbrega G. Clínica e terapêutica da doença de Chagas. *Memórias do Instituto Oswaldo Cruz.* 1948; 46: 473-529.

[31] Laranja F. Chagas' Disease: a Clinical, Epidemiologic and Pathologic Study. *Circulation.* 1956; 14: 1035-60.

[32] Kropf SP. En busca de la enfermedad del Brasil: los médicos del interior y los estudios sobre el mal de Chagas (1935-1956). In: Carbonetti A, González-Leandri R., editors. *Historias de Salud y Enfermedad en América Latina, Siglos XIX y XX.* Córdoba: Universidad Nacional de Córdoba, Conicet; 2008.

[33] World Health Organization. Chagas' Disease: report of a Study Group. Geneva; 1960 (*WHO Technical Report Series No. 202*).

[34] Escobar A. Encountering Development: the making and unmaking of the Third World. Princeton, New Jersey: *Princeton University Press*; 1995.

[35] Winslow CEA. *Lo que Cuesta la Enfermedad y lo que Vale la Salud. Washington: Organización Mundial de la Salud*, Oficina Sanitaria Panamericana; mayo 1955.

[36] Kropf SP. Carlos Chagas: science, health, and national debate in Brazil. *The Lancet.* May 2011, 377, 1740-1741. Available from: *http://download.thelancet.com/pdfs/journals/lancet/PIIS0140673611607216.pdf*

In: Chagas Disease   ISBN: 978-1-62808-681-2
Editors: F. R. Gadelha, E.d.F. Peloso   © 2013 Nova Science Publishers, Inc.

Chapter II

Trypanosoma cruzi, the Etiologic Agent of Chagas Disease

Fernanda Ramos Gadelha

Departamento de Bioquímica, Instituto de Biologia
Universidade Estadual de Campinas, Campinas-SP, Brazil

Abstract

Trypanosoma cruzi causes a relevant human pathology, Chagas disease. Currently, the drugs employed in treatment are unsatisfactory, there is no vaccine and a large number of people are either infected or living in endemic areas. The search for new targets in the development of specific chemotherapies has led to in-depth research of parasite cell biology. The cell biology of *T. cruzi* is remarkable in several aspects. The life cycle of *T. cruzi* is complex, involving a vertebrate and an invertebrate host, four distinct developmental forms, trypomastigotes (bloodstream and metacyclic), amastigotes and epimastigotes that inhabit distinct environments. The heterogeneity among strains has been the Achilles' heel in the development of improved therapies. In addition to the structures and organelles that are present in other eukaryotic cells, *T. cruzi* possess several unique ones such as the glycosome, the flagellar pocket, the kinetoplast and even some structures and organelles present in only one evolutionary form such as the reservosome in the epimastigote stage. This chapter will review the most peculiar features of the parasite with the intent to correlate the structure and function of the organelles to their relevant adaptive and survival advantage in each environment of each stage of the life cycle of *T. cruzi*.

Introduction

Trypanosoma cruzi, the causative agent of Chagas disease, is a flagellate protozoan parasite belonging to the Sarcomastigophora Phylum; Zoomastigophora class; Kinetoplastida order; Trypanosomatidade family [1]. This family encompasses important genera of species that cause human disease such as Leishmania, Phytomonas, Crithidia, and Trypanosoma, among others. *T. cruzi* belongs to the Stercoraria group of the Trypanosoma genus, which consists of parasites that develop along the digestive track of invertebrate hosts and are released in their infective form in the vector's feces [2].

T. cruzi comprises a pool of isolates, or strains, that display significant heterogeneity regarding their biological parameters: degree of virulence in laboratory animals and humans [3]; tissue tropism [4]; biochemical features such as those in oxidative metabolism [5, 6], antioxidant defenses and susceptibility to drugs [7, 8]; and genetic variation [reviewed in 9]. This intra-species heterogeneity could modulate parasite pathogenicity, survival and adaptability [3, 5, 10]. *T. cruzi* is a diploid organism that multiplies by binary division, but genetic exchange with homologous recombination can occur [reviewed in 9]. The differences in symptoms and geographical variations in the prevalence of the clinical forms of Chagas disease and its distinct response to treatment have been attributed to the diversity in the *T. cruzi* population. It is important to note that the environmental, nutritional and immunological aspects of the host may also play important roles.

Over the years, in an attempt to characterize the role of parasite diversity in the epidemiology and pathogenesis of Chagas disease, different approaches have been used to type and group strains of *T. cruzi*. One such approach, isoenzyme pattern analysis, led to the establishment of three groups, designated zymodemes 1, 2 and 3 [11]. Another method using DNA markers clustered the *T. cruzi* population into lineages 1, 2 and hybrids [12]. A more recent method, multilocus genotyping, *i.e.* the genetic constitution of a given strain based on different DNA regions, sorted the strains into discrete typing units (DTU) defined as "sets of stocks that are genetically more related to each other than to any other stock and that are identifiable by common genetic, molecular or immunological markers called tags" [13, 14]. Six DTUs were identified on the basis of multilocus enzyme electrophoresis and random amplified polymorphic DNA characterization [15]. Further comparison among the genomes from isolates of various DTUs will improve our knowledge on parasite pathogenicity and epidemiologic features.

Life Cycle

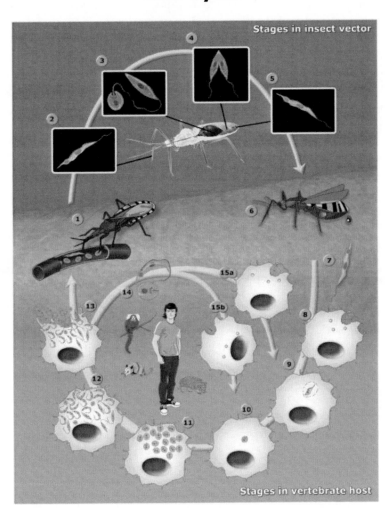

Figure 1. Trypanosoma cruzi life cycle [reproduced from 20; doi:10.1371/journal.pntd. 0001749.g001].

The life cycle of *T. cruzi* was elucidated by Carlos Chagas [16], who revealed that the parasite has a complex life cycle that alternates among a vertebrate and an invertebrate host, taking turns between replicative and non-replicative and infective and non-infective forms. *T. cruzi* can infect a wide range of mammals such as human beings, sylvan and domestic animals as well as invertebrates such as triatomine hematophagous insect vectors. The parasite has four morphologically and biochemically distinct developmental stages during its life cycle: in the invertebrate host, the epimastigotes, (replicative and non-infective) and the metacyclic trypomastigotes (infectious and non-replicative); in the vertebrate host, trypomastigotes and amastigotes (both infective) [17], but the former is non-replicative, while the latter is replicative.

Figure 1 shows the life cycle of *T. cruzi* [reviewed in 18]. The vectors illustrated belong to the Reduviidae family (Triatominae sub-family) and are blood-sucking insects popularly called "kissing bugs" because the bite is often on or near the face. The "kissing bug" can become infected after taking up blood from an infected mammal (Figure 1, #1) that contains bloodstream trypomastigotes, and up to 10% of amastigotes (Figure 1, #2). In the midgut of the vector, trypomastigotes differentiate into amastigotes (Figure 1, #3), which swell and extend their flagella and can be visualized once their flagella are beating. At this point, flagellated amastigotes are sometimes referred to as spheromastigotes. Next, this form enters the epimastigote stage. The epimastigotes multiply by binary division (Figure 1, #4), and after attaching to the cuticle of the hindgut wall via the tip of their flagella, they differentiate into metacyclic trypomastigotes (Figure 1, #5). This process is called metacyclogenesis, takes approximately 48 h and appears to be triggered by the interaction between the flagellum and the substrate to which it attaches. Nutritional stress in the insect's gut is also capable of inducing this process [19]. After detaching from this cuticle of the hindgut wall, metacyclic trypomastigotes are eliminated with the feces of the vector upon defecation following a blood meal (Figure 1, #6).

The parasite (Figure 1, #7) is not capable of penetrating intact skin; it only infects the vertebrate host either through the bite wound, after rubbing/scratching by the host, or directly through a mucosal membrane. Once in the bloodstream, *T. cruzi* can infect a variety of cells including macrophages, muscle and epithelial cells. In macrophages (Figure 1 #8), the parasite is internalized through phagocytosis and the lysosome fuses with it, leading to the formation of the endocytic vacuole, also known as the parasitophorous vacuole (Figure 1, #9). There are different mechanisms by which the parasite can penetrate into the host cell [reviewed in 21], but no matter what pathway is followed, the parasite resides within a parasitophorous vacuole [22]. The metacyclic forms transform into amastigotes, (Figure 1, #10), which multiply by binary division in the cytoplasm of the cell (Figure 1, #11) after lysis of the parasitophorous vacuole by enzymes secreted by the parasite [23]. The amastigotes then transform into blood stream trypomastigotes (Figure 1, #12) that burst out of the cell (Figure 1, #13) and can infect neighboring cells by a process similar to the one described for the metacyclic trypomastigotes. They can also gain access to the bloodstream where they can reach other host tissues and re-start the life-cycle (Figure 1, #14-15). Some amastigotes are also released during cell lysis and can infect cells, albeit by a different process than trypomastigotes. Also represented in Figure 1 are the main animal reservoirs involved in the maintenance of *T. cruzi* in the domestic and peridomestic environment [20, reviewed in 18, 21]. In Chapter III, the diversity among vector species, the reservoirs and the mode of transmission of Chagas disease will be further discussed.

Developmental Stages

In 1909, Carlos Chagas made the first morphologic descriptions of *T. cruzi* developmental stages found in the vertebrate and invertebrate hosts. The kinetoplast is a fibrous network of DNA located in the mitochondrion that constitutes 20-25% of the total parasite DNA [24], assumes different sizes and shapes according to the developmental stage and whose relative position in relation to the cell nucleus and the emergence of the flagellum allows for the characterization of the different forms of the parasite:

(1) **Trypomastigotes** are elongated and approximately 0.25 mm long [22], with the kinetoplast at the posterior end of the parasite with the nucleus; the flagellar pocket, from which the flagellum emerges, is located at the posterior region of the parasite near the kinetoplast; the flagellum attaches along the body of the parasite and is free at the anterior end of the parasite [22, 24, 25]. Morphologically, aside from the differences in the cell surface membrane, addressed below, the trypomastigotes and metacyclic trypomastigotes appear to be structurally similar.

In the laboratory, metacyclic trypomastigotes are obtained upon incubation of epimastigotes in triatomine artificial urine (TAU), a medium that mimics the composition of the insect's urine and is supplemented with amino acids and glucose. Under these conditions, parasites adhere to the flask and undergo differentiation [26]. Trypomastigotes released from infected cells adhered to the walls of the flask are collected from the extracellular medium. The tissue-derived trypomastigotes are then cultivated in culture medium rich in amino acids and vitamins, such as Dulbecco´s Modified Eagle Medium (DMEM) supplemented with 2% fetal calf serum [27]. Infected and non-infected cells are kept in an incubator at 37°C with 5% CO_2.

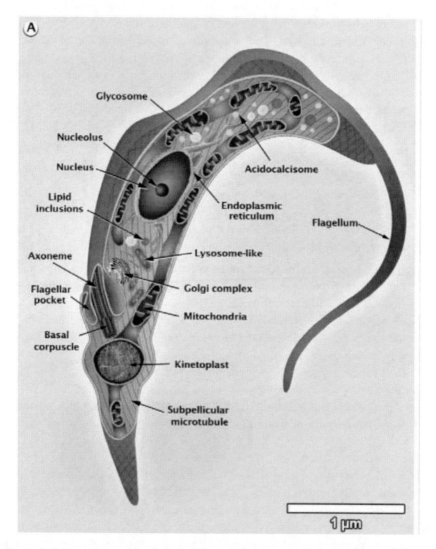

Figure 2. Schematic representation of *Trypanosoma cruzi* trypomastigotes organelles. [reproduced from 20; doi:10.1371/journal.pntd.0001749.g004]

(2) **Amastigotes** are round and 0.03-0.05 mm in diameter, and the kinetoplast is localized anterior to the nucleus and has a short flagellum that often stays inside the flagellar pocket [22].

In the laboratory, these forms can be obtained from infected cells after homogenization and separation of the free parasites from cell debris via centrifugation [28].

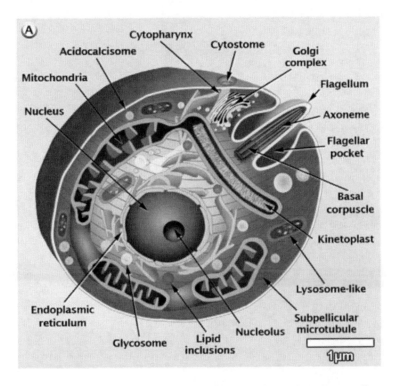

Figure 3. Schematic representation of *Trypanosoma cruzi* amastigotes organelles. [reproduced from 20; doi:10.1371/journal.pntd.0001749.g002].

(3) **Epimastigotes** are elongated, 0.20-0.40mm long, with the kinetoplast and the flagellar pocket found anterior to the nucleus [22, 24].

In the laboratory, epimastigotes are grown at 28 °C in Liver Infusion Tryptose (LIT) medium containing 20 mg/L of hemin and 10% fetal calf serum [29]. Hemin must be provided in the culture medium, as it is essential for *T. cruzi* and constitutes a key molecule in many biological reactions such as oxygen consumption by the mitochondrion, a process mediated by heme-containing proteins such as cytochromes.

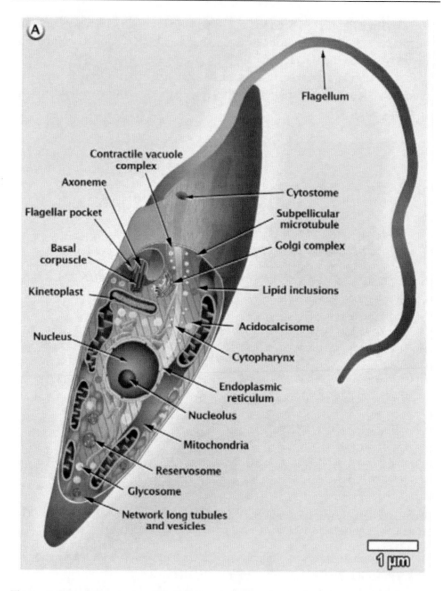

Figure 4. Schematic representation of *Trypanosoma cruzi* epimastigotes organelles. [reproduced from 20; doi:10.1371/journal.pntd.0001749.g003].

Cell Biology

In addition to the organelles present in an ordinary eukaryotic cell, *T. cruzi* has peculiar ones. Additionally, some already known differences in eukaryotic structures make not only *T. cruzi* but also the trypanosomatids in general unique eukaryotes. The interesting features of *T. cruzi* cell biology will be discussed below.

1. Cell Surface

The composition and structure of the cell surface is fundamental for the interaction of the parasite with the host. The cell surface can be considered to include the lipid bilayer and associated components that face the extracellular medium and form the glycocalyx, also known as the surface coat [30]. The composition of the glycocalyx is characteristic of each differential stage and includes carbohydrates (e.g., sialic acid) associated with peripheral or integrated proteins (glycoproteins (gp)) such as mucins or lipids (glycolipids) that project to the outer side of the cell. The importance and the diversity of the cell surface composition can be demonstrated through *T. cruzi* oral route experiments. Metacyclic trypomastigotes express gp82, which plays an important role in the establishment of infection through its ability to bind to gastric mucin present in the mucus layer that protects the stomach mucosa [31]. Culture-derived trypomastigotes do not present gp82 and rarely infect mice by the oral route [32], but rather express Tc85-11 that binds laminin, making the dissemination of the parasite through the organism easier [33]. Interestingly, metacyclic trypomastigotes are resistant to treatment at acidic pH with pepsin, a digestive enzyme, while blood trypomastigotes are highly sensitive to this treatment. Epimastigotes are killed by the complement system when exposed to fresh human serum [34]; their cell surface lack gp82 or Tc85-11 [35] and is made of peculiar glycolipids and glycoproteins anchored to the membrane through phosphatidylinositol, making these cells resistant to proteases and glycosidases [25]. Taking all this into account, it is clear that cell surface composition plays a fundamental role in enabling the parasite to reach the target cell and to survive within the host.

Sialic acids are fundamental for parasite survival in the mammalian host, but *T. cruzi* is not capable of performing *de novo* synthesis of these molecules [36] and therefore must import them from the host. Transialidases (TS) are present in the cell surface of *T. cruzi* and mediate the transfer of sialic acids, present in proteins of the extracellular environment, to the mucins of the parasite. This sialylation of the parasite helps to protect it from the action of antibodies, enabling it to reach the bloodstream and spread. TS also play a role in cell attachment, invasion and parasite escape from the parasitophorous vacuole [25, 37].

2. The Cytoskeleton

The cytoskeleton is made of sub-pellicular microtubules distributed, except for the flagellar pocket region, throughout the parasite body [30]. In trypanosomatids, the association between the plasma membrane and the sub-peculliar microtubules is tighter than in other eukaryotic cells [22], making it difficult to disrupt the cell through conventional methods. This has been a drawback in the study of intracellular organelles of the parasite. Digitonin, a steroid glycoside, has been used to selectively permeabilize trypanosomatid plasma membranes without affecting the structure and function of mitochondria, endoplasmic reticulum and acidocalcisomes [38]. The effect of digitonin is mainly due to the formation of insoluble complexes with cholesterol; because the plasma membrane has a high cholesterol/phospholipid ratio in relation to that of intracellular organelles, it allows for the selective permeabilization of the plasma membrane [38]. The use of digitonin made possible the study of trypanosomatid energy-linked functions and calcium homeostasis; it was also a powerful tool in the determination of the intracellular localization of proteins.

Interestingly, it has been recently proposed that in addition to a structural role in these cells, the cytoskeleton proteins may directly participate in the signaling pathway that is activated during parasite attachment to the host cell [39].

3. The Flagellum and the Flagellar Pocket

In *T. cruzi*, as well as in all the members of the Trypanosomatidae family, the flagellum emerges from the flagellar pocket, an invagination of the plasma membrane that establishes direct continuity with the flagellum membrane [22]. Interestingly, the plasma membrane, the membrane lining the flagellum and the flagellar pocket have unique protein and possibly lipid compositions that contribute to distinct functions [40]. There are significant differences among the evolutionarily distinct plasma membranes, each made of a lipid bilayer with differing degrees of associated proteins, such as permeases, responsible for the uptake of nutrients. In addition to being involved in parasite attachment to the endothelium of the insect vector and possibly in sensing the environment, the flagellum is responsible for parasite movement by wave-like beats of the microtubule-based flagellar axoneme. Further, the flagellar pocket is responsible for the uptake of macromolecules via receptor-mediated endocytosis, exocytosis and delivery of proteins to the cell surface and the extracellular medium [22, 25, 40].

Similar to other flagella, the flagellum of *T. cruzi* is surrounded by a flagellar membrane containing a typical axonema with a pattern of nine peripheral microtubule doublets and one central doublet [30] emerging laterally in trypomastigotes and epimastigotes [22]. In addition to the axoneme, the epimastigotes and trypomastigotes flagellum has a complex structure called the paraflagellar rod (PFR) [25]. The PFR is made of a complex array of filaments linked to the axoneme and is composed of a large number of proteins. Two of these proteins, PFR 1 and 2, are highly antigenic and constitute targets for vaccine and diagnostic kit development [30].

The flagellar membrane has a unique protein and lipid composition. It is rich in lipid rafts, platforms known to organize transmembrane signaling events. Lipid rafts also have many proteins associated with them that either enrich the flagellar membrane or are completely restricted to it. Many of these proteins are suggested to be involved in sensing and signaling, widening the role of the flagella beyond motility and host cell invasion [41]. Calcium-binding proteins that appear to be involved in signal transduction mediated by changes in intracellular calcium levels are also present in the flagellar membrane [40].

Because the membranes covering the cell body and the flagellum have physical contact to one other at the point where the flagellum emerges, the flagellar pocket can be considered as a special extracellular compartment in some way isolated from the extracellular medium [22]. As discussed, it is a highly specialized component of the plasma membrane that is designed for uptake and secretion of molecules required by or released from the parasite [40].

4. Cytostome and Reservosome

Epimastigotes and amastigotes have a specialized structure known as the cytostome-cytopharynx complex. It appears as a funnel-shaped structure formed from a deep invagination of the plasma membrane. The opening of this complex is called the cytostome [22]. This structure penetrates deep into the cytoplasm toward the nucleus and, in association with the flagellar pocket membrane, appears to play an important role in the nutrition of the parasite [42]; pinocytosis and 85% of the endocytic activity occurs in the cytostome [43]. Endocytic vesicles bud from the flagellar pocket or the cytostome, the two sites for macromolecule ingestion in epimastigotes, and fuse with a branched vesicular tubular network that composes early endosomes. Afterwards, the cargo of the endocytic vesicles is delivered to the reservosomes, which are localized at the posterior region of the protozoan [30], an organelle found exclusively in epimastigotes [22]. In amastigotes and trypomastigotes, similar organelles that shared some reservosome features were found, but they differ from reservosomes in their ability to store external macromolecules [30].

Each epimastigote has several reservosomes, mainly located in the posterior region of the cell [30] surrounded by a unit membrane, with a morphology that can vary according to growth conditions and parasite strain [22] and occupy approximately 6% of the total cell volume [44].

Although they also concentrate lysosomal hydrolases, reservosomes are acidic organelles whose main function is to store macromolecules. Cruzipain, cysteine protease and the main epimastigote protease, is also found inside the reservosome. Consequently, reservosomes, and related ones found not only in amastigotes but also in trypomastigotes, were suggested to be considered as lysosomal-related organelles because they share many features as those described in mammalian lysosomes [30].

Reservosomes gradually vanish during differentiation into trypo-mastigotes, i.e. metacyclogenesis, raising the possibility that the nutrients stored in the reservosomes are used as an energy source during this process [44]. In the reverse process, during the transformation of trypomastigotes into epimastigotes in the insect vector, new reservosomes appear to originate from the Golgi complex at the anterior region of the parasite and then migrate towards the posterior region [45].

5. Acidocalcisomes

These organelles are acidic, calcium-storage organelles first described in trypanosomes but later found in different organisms. The membrane composition is unique, differs from other organelle membranes and contains several pumps, exchangers and at least one channel (aquaporin) involved in the uptake of several ions and water [46]. These organelles are randomly distributed in the cells and are present in greater numbers in amastigotes than in epimastigotes and trypomastigotes [25].

Acidocalcisomes mainly store phosphorous, both as inorganic pyrophosphate (PPi) and polyphosphate (poly P), a linear chain of several to many hundreds of phosphate residues; poly P in prokaryotes has been linked with virulence [47]; cations such as calcium (at high levels), magnesium, potassium, sodium combined with poly P and basic amino acids, arginine and lysine [48].

In addition to functioning as a storage organelle, other functions have been attributed to acidocalcisomes, such as pH homeostasis and osmoregulation in conjunction with the contractile vacuole [48, 49]. *T. cruzi* faces extreme changes in its osmotic environments during its life cycle, and the release of ions and osmolytes, such as potassium and amino acids, could aid the parasite in adjusting cell volume after an osmotic stress induced during transmission [49]. Therefore, these organelles and their major component, poly P, are essential for responding to different stress conditions; lower levels of poly P are associated with a decreased ability to respond to osmotic or nutritional stresses as well as decreased virulence in vitro and in vivo [46].

6. Glycosomes

Glycosomes are spherical structures with a homogenous matrix surrounded by a unit membrane [30]. The first six enzymes of the glycolytic pathway are located in the glycosome [50], so there is cooperation among the cytosol, mitochondrion and glycosomes in energy metabolism. One possible explanation for the compartmentalization of these enzymes is the lack of allosteric regulation of hexokinase and phosphofructokinase, which would result in glycolytic flux being controlled at the level of glucose uptake into the glycosome [51]. Additionally, the enzymes involved in the pentose phosphate pathway, another possible pathway for glucose metabolism, appear to be present, at least partially, in glycosomes to produce NADPH and ribulose-5-phosphate for other enzymatic reactions that occur inside this organelle [52].

7. Nucleus

The structural organization of the nucleus appears to be similar to other eukaryotic cells. Although, in trypomastigotes, the nucleus is elongated and localized in the central portion of the cell and it is slightly spherical in epimastigotes and amastigotes. The chromosomes are difficult to distinguish because they do not condense at any stage of the life cycle [22, 25]. Specific genes are differentially expressed during the life cycle, which gives the parasite plasticity to overcome the challenges of living in such different environments [53]. Interestingly, genome-wide studies showed that epigenetic regulation might play a very important role in gene expression in trypanosomatids [54].

T. cruzi has many unusual genetic features, such as intron-less genes, polycistronic transcription and regulation of gene expression by post-transcriptional mechanisms. The protein coding genes are organized into long, strand-specific, polycistronic clusters. Polycistronic primary transcripts are processed into monogenic mRNAs by means of 5'-end trans-splicing (i.e. addition of the spliced leader sequence) and 3'-end polyadenylation reactions [54, 55]. Genetic exchange occurs in both *T. brucei* and *T. cruzi* [56].

In the genome of *T. cruzi*, over 50% of it consists of repeated sequences such as retrotransposons and genes for large families of surface molecules, which include trans-sialidase and mucins, among others. Further, analysis of the *T. cruzi* genome imply differences from other eukaryotes in DNA repair and the initiation of replication, and reflect their unusual mitochondrial DNA [56].

8. Mitochondrion and the Kinetoplast

T. cruzi has only one highly ramified mitochondrion per cell that occupies one third of parasite cell volume [25, 30]. The mitochondrion of *T. cruzi* shares with its mammalian counterpart some features such as the inner and outer membranes and the presence of DNA, cristae and a number of enzymes. As discussed above, digitonin has been used for the selective permeabilization of the plasma membrane and, in so doing, has allowed for study of the organelles in situ; much of the knowledge on how mitochondria work in *T. cruzi* came from these studies. Recently, another protocol was standardized where cells subjected to abrasion in a chilled mortar in the presence of glass beads followed by differential centrifugation allowed us to obtain a mitochondria fraction [57].

Currently, it is clear that in addition to being the major site of ATP generation, the mitochondrion is also a source of signaling molecules involved in apoptosis, the cell cycle and proliferation [58]. Among the signaling molecules, reactive oxygen species (ROS) stand out. They are produced as byproducts of the mitochondrial respiratory chain [reviewed in 6]. To avoid damage, the mitochondrion, as well as other organelles besides the cytoplasm, is equipped, to some extent, with an efficient antioxidant system.

Mitochondrial DNA, or K-DNA, is located within the mitochondrial matrix, perpendicular to the axis of the flagellum; it is always located close to the basal body connected by filamentous structures [30]. K-DNA molecules are organized as associated mini- and maxicircles. The minicircles are present in a large number and encode guide RNAs that modify maxicircle transcripts by extensive uridylate insertion or deletion, a process known as RNA editing [30, reviewed in 59]. Maxicircles are structurally and functionally analogous to the mitochondrial DNA in higher eukaryotes that encodes rRNAs and the subunits of respiratory complexes [24, 30].

9. Host-Parasite Interactions

To establish infection, a great variety of molecules from the parasite and the host may play an important role. The heterogeneity of the *T. cruzi* population is an important factor, but other parameters should be considered as described below.

In the invertebrate host - epimastigotes attach to the perimicrovillar membranes of the cells of the posterior midgut of the invertebrate host; this step is essential for the metacyclogenesis process to occur. Attachment involves a process of cell-to-cell recognition with the involvement of sugar residues exposed on the surface of both interacting cells [30, 60]. The digestion of blood in the vector generates free radicals due to the presence of iron-containing hemoglobin, which is highly susceptible to oxidation [25]. Interestingly, hemin, the product of hemoglobin degradation, is capable of increasing the proliferation of epimastigotes but can induce ROS-induced damage at higher concentrations [61]. To prevent damage, the parasite has an efficient antioxidant system in which variation in the expression of proteins involved in this system depends on the strain and on the phase of parasite growth [7].

In the vertebrate host - According to de Souza et al [21], the first steps in host-parasite consist of three stages: (1) adhesion and recognition of molecules on the parasite or host cell surface; (2) signaling; and (3) invasion. A lot is known about which parasite molecules are involved, but not much information is available regarding which host molecules are important for this interplay. Parasite molecules, including glycoproteins such as mucins, have been implicated in the process of adhesion and recognition; the major surface glycoproteins of trypomastigotes include Tc85, an 85 kDa glycoprotein, and gp82 and gp 35/50 expressed on the surface of metacyclic trypomastigotes. However, no surface component involved in adhesion or recognition has yet been identified in amastigotes [21].

After binding and recognition, the next step is signaling, which culminates with cell invasion. Both parasite and host molecules are involved in this process. Three distinct mechanisms are postulated to be used by the trypomastigote to signal and invade host cells: (1) the lysosome-dependent pathway, which is initiated by the exocytosis of lysosomes in the plasma membrane and is regulated by Ca^{2+}; (2) the actin-dependent pathway, in which trypomastigotes penetrate a host cell through a plasma membrane expansion that ends with the formation of the parasitophorous vacuole to which lysosomes fuse; and (3) the lysosome-independent pathway, in which the parasite enters the cell through membrane invaginations [21]. Independent of the invasion mechanism, the parasite ends up inside a parasitophorous vacuole. Ca^{2+} plays a significant role in the recognition process; a transient increase in intracellular concentrations, both in the host cell and parasite, is fundamental for parasite invasion [62]. Amastigotes use the actin-dependent phagocytic pathway for internalization [63].

A novel mechanism to explain parasite interaction with the host is vesicle release by *T. cruzi*. These vesicles contain major surface components that are involved in parasite adhesion to and invasion of host cells as well as members of the gp85/trans-sialidase glycoprotein superfamily, mucins, and proteases, among others, that are important in evading host immune mechanisms. Parasite-shed vesicles could be acting as messengers to prime host cells for invasion either by interacting with host cell surface components or being internalized, somehow preparing the host cell for the incoming trypanosome. These vesicles are virulence factors and should be further studied to understand the pathogenesis of Chagas disease [reviewed in 64].

Conclusion

Carlos Chagas made the first descriptions of the morphology of different evolutionary forms of *T. cruzi* in 1909. Since then, in-depth studies have aimed to not only understand the changes that occur in cell biology throughout the life cycle of *T. cruzi* but also establish the correlation among the structure, function and relevance of the intracellular organelles for each particular developmental form. It is noteworthy that this parasite has unique features of cell biology such as the presence of only one mitochondrion per cell, the presence of organelles such as the reservosome in the epimastigote stage but not in other stages, which seem to be important for the metacyclogenesis process, the unique composition of the plasma membrane in each stage, the heterogeneity among parasite strains and other interesting features. Although substantial research has been conducted, there are still gaps, and future studies will guide us toward a better understanding of the tools employed by *T. cruzi* that allow for its survival and adaption in different hosts. In the end, this will provide us with a framework of possible targets for the development of more specific therapies.

References

[1]　Teixeira AR, Nascimento RJ, Sturm NR. Evolution and pathology in chagas disease: a review. *Mem Inst Oswaldo Cruz.* 2006; 101(5): 463-91.

[2]　Brener Z. *Trypanosoma cruzi*: morfologia e ciclo evolutivo. In: Dias JCP and Coura JR (Eds). Clínica e Terapêutica da doença de Chagas. Uma abordagem para o clínico geral. *Fiocruz Ed., Rio de Janeiro.* 1997; 25-32.

[3]　Rimoldi A, Tomé Alves R, Ambrósio DL, Fernandes MZ, Martinez I, De Araújo RF, Cicarelli RM, Da Rosa JA. Morphological, biological and molecular characterization of three strains of *Trypanosoma cruzi* Chagas, 1909 (Kinetoplastida, Trypanosomatidae) isolated from *Triatoma sordida* (Stal) 1859 (Hemiptera, Reduviidae) and a domestic cat. *Parasitol.* 2012;139(1): 37-44.

[4]　Melo RC, Brener Z. Tissue tropism of different *Trypanosoma cruzi* strains. *J Parasitol.* 1978; 64(3): 475-82.

[5]   Engel JC, Doyle PS, Dvorak JA. Isolate-dependent differences in the oxidative metabolism of *Trypanosoma cruzi* epimastigotes. *Mol Biochem Parasitol.* 1990; 39(1): 69-76.

[6]   Silva TM, Peloso EF, Vitor SC, Ribeiro LH, Gadelha FR. O_2 consumption rates along the growth curve: new insights into *Trypanosoma cruzi* mitochondrial respiratory chain. *J Bioenerg Biomembr.* 2011; 43(4): 409-17.

[7]   Peloso EF, Gonçalves CC, Silva TM, Ribeiro LH, Piñeyro MD, Robello C, Gadelha FR. Tryparedoxin peroxidases and superoxide dismutases expression as well as ROS release are related to *Trypanosoma cruzi* epimastigotes growth phases. *Arch Biochem Biophys.* 2012; 520(2): 117-22.

[8]   Murta SM, Gazzinelli RT, Brener Z, Romanha AJ. Molecular characterization of susceptible and naturally resistant strains of *Trypanosoma cruzi* to benznidazole and nifurtimox. *Mol Biochem Parasitol.* 1998; 93(2): 203-14.

[9]   Macedo AM, Machado CR, Oliveira RP, Pena SD. *Trypanosoma cruzi*: genetic structure of populations and relevance of genetic variability to the pathogenesis of chagas disease. *Mem Inst Oswaldo Cruz.* 2004; 99(1): 1-12.

[10] Brisse S, Barnabé C, Bañuls AL, Sidibé I, Noël S, Tibayrenc M. A phylogenetic analysis of the *T. cruzi* genome project CL Brener reference strain by multilocus enzyme electrophoresis and multiprimer random amplified polymorphic DNA fingerprinting. *Mol Biochem Parasitol.* 1998; 9: 253–63.

[11] Miles MA, Souza A, Povoa M, Shaw JJ, Lainson R, Toye PJ. lsozymic heterogeneity of *Trypanosoma cruzi* in the first autochtonous patients with Chagas' disease in Amazonian Brazil. *Nature.* 1978; 272: 819-21.

[12] Souto RP, Fernandes O, Macedo AM, Campbell DA, Zingales B. DNA markers define two major phylogenetic lineages of *Trypanosoma cruzi*. *Mol Biochem Parasitol.* 1996; 83: 141- 52.

[13] Tibayrenc M. Integrated genetic epidemiology of infectious diseases: the Chagas model. *Mem Inst Oswaldo Cruz.* 1998; 93(5): 577-80.

[14] Tibayrenc M, Ayala FJ. The clonal theory of parasitic protozoa: 12 years on. *Trends Parasitol.* 2002; 18(9): 405-10.

[15] Brisse S, Dujardin JC, Tibayrenc M. Identification of six *Trypanosoma cruzi* lineages by sequence-characterised amplified region markers. *Mol Biochem Parasitol.* 2000; 111(1): 95-105.

[16] Chagas C. (1909). Nova tripanozomase humana. Estudos sobre a morfologia e o ciclo evolutivo do *Schizotrypanum cruzi* n. gen. sp, agente etiológico de nova entidade mórbida do homem. *Mem Inst Oswaldo Cruz.* 1909; 1: 159–218.

[17] de Carvalho TU, de Souza W. Infectivity of amastigotes of *Trypanosoma cruzi. Rev Inst Med Trop São Paulo.* 1986; 28(4): 205-12.

[18] Tyler KM, Engman DM. The life cycle of *Trypanosoma cruzi* revisited. *Int J Parasitol.* 2001; 31(5-6): 472-81.

[19] Wainszelbaum MJ, Belaunzarán ML, Lammel EM, Florin-Christensen M, Florin-Christensen J, Isola EL. Free fatty acids induce cell differentiation to infective forms in *Trypanosoma cruzi. Biochem J.* 2003; 375(Pt 3): 705-12.

[20] Teixeira DE, Benchimol M, Crepaldi PH, de Souza W. Interactive multimedia to teach the life cycle of *Trypanosoma cruzi*, the causative agent of Chagas disease. *PLoS Negl Trop Dis.* 2012; 6(8): e1749.

[21] de Souza W, de Carvalho TMU, Barrias ES. Review on *Trypanosoma cruzi*: Host Cell Interaction. *Int J Cell Biology.* 2010; 2010 Article ID 295394, 18 pages.

[22] De Souza W. Basic cell biology of *Trypanosoma cruzi. Curr Pharm Des.* 2002; 8(4): 269-85.

[23] de Carvalho TM, de Souza W. Early events related with the behaviour of *Trypanosoma cruzi* within an endocytic vacuole in mouse peritoneal macrophages. *Cell Struct Funct.* 1989; 14(4): 383-92.

[24] Brener Z. *Trypanosoma cruzi*: taxonomy, mosphology and life cycle. In: *Chagas Disease (American Trypanosomiasis): its impact on transfusion and clinical medicine.* Wendel S, Brener Z, Camargo ME, Rassi A (Eds). ISBT BRAZIL'92, São Paulo, Brazil. 1992: 13-29.

[25] de Souza W. Study by transmission electron microscopy (on line). Available from: http: *http://www.fiocruz.br/chagas_eng/cgi/cgilua.exe/ sys/start.htm?sid=13*

[26] Contreras VT, Salles JM, Thomas N, Morel CM, Goldenberg S. In vitro differentiation of *Trypanosoma cruzi* under chemically defined conditions. *Mol Biochem Parasitol.* 1985; 16: 315-27.

[27] Gadelha FR, Gonçalves CC, Mattos EC, Alves MJ, Piñeyro MD, Robello C, Peloso EF. Release of the cytosolic tryparedoxin peroxidase into the incubation medium and a different profile of cytosolic and mitochondrial peroxiredoxin expression in H_2O_2-treated *Trypanosoma cruzi* tissue culture-derived trypomastigotes. *Exp Parasitol.* 2013; 133(3): 287-93.

[28] Abuin G, Freitas-Junior LHG, Colli W, Alves MJM, Schenkman S.
      Expression of trans-sialidase and 85-kDa glycoprotein genes in
      Trypanosoma cruzi is differentially regulated at the post-transcriptional
      level by labile protein factors. *J Biol Chem.* 1999; 274: 13041–7.

[29] Castellani O, Ribeiro L, Fernandes F. Differentiation of *Trypanosoma
      cruzi* in culture. *J Protozool.* 1967; 14: 447–51.

[30] Souza, W. Structural organization of *Trypanosoma cruzi. Mem Inst
      Oswaldo Cruz.* 2009; 104 (Suppl. I): 89-100.

[31] Staquicini DI, Martins RMM, Macedo S, Sasso GRS, Atayde VD,
      Juliano MA, Toshida N. Role of gp82 in the selective binding to gastric
      mucin during infection with *Trypanosoma cruzi. PLoS Negl Trop Dis.*
      2010; 4(3): e613

[32] Hoft DF, Farrar PL, Kratz-Owens K, Shaffer D. Gastric invasion by
      Trypanosoma cruzi and induction of protective mucosal immune
      responses. *Infect Immun.* 1996; 64: 3800–10.

[33] [33] Giordano R. Fouts D, Tewari D, Colli W, Manning J, Alves, MJM.
      (1999) Cloning of a surface membrane glycoprotein specific for the
      infective form of *Trypanosoma cruzi* having adhesive properties to
      laminin. J Biol Chem. 1999; 274: 3461–8.

[34] Ameisen JC, Idzioerk T, Billaut-Mulot O, Tissier JP, Potentier A,
      Ouaissi A. (1995) Apoptosis in a unicellular eukaryote (*Trypanosoma
      cruzi*): implications for the evolutionary origin and role of programmed
      cell death in the control of cell proliferation, differentiation and survival.
      Cell Death Differ. 1995; 2: 285–300.

[35] Cortez C, Yoshida N, Bahia D, Sobreira TJ. Structural basis of the
      interaction of a *Trypanosoma cruzi* surface molecule implicated in oral
      infection with host cells and gastric mucin. *PLoS One.* 2012; 7(7):
      e42153.

[36] Previato JO, Andrade AF, Pessolani MC, Mendonca-Previato L (1985)
      Incorporation of sialic acid into *Trypanosoma cruzi* macromolecules. A
      proposal for a new metabolic route. *Mol Biochem Parasitol.* 1985; 16:
      85–96.

[37] Buschiazzo A, Muiá R, Larrieux N, Pitcovsky T, Mucci J, Campetella
      O. *Trypanosoma cruzi* trans-sialidase in complex with a neutralizing
      antibody: structure/function studies towards the rational design of
      inhibitors. *PLoS Pathog.* 2012; 8(1): e1002474.

[38] Rodrigues CO, Catisti R, Ueymura SA, Vercesi AE, Lira R, Rodriguez
      C, Urbina JU, Docampo R. The sterol composition of *Trypanosoma
      cruzi* changes after growth in different culture media and results in

different sensitivity to digitonin-permeabilization. *J Euk Microbiol.* 2001; 48(5): 588-94.

[39]   Mattos EC, Schumacher RI, Colli W, Alves MJM. Adhesion of *Trypanosoma cruzi* trypomastigotes to fibronectin or laminin modifies tubulin and paraflagellar rod protein phosphorylation. *PloS One.* 2012; 7(10): e46767.

[40]   Landfear SM, Ignatushchenko M. The flagellum and flagellar pocket of trypanosomatids. *Mol Biochem Parasitol.* 2001; 115: 1-17.

[41]   Maric D, Epting CL, Engman DM. Composition and sensory function of the trypanosome flagellar membrane. *Curr Opin Microbiol.* 2010; 13(4): 466–72.

[42]   Okuda K, Esteva M, Segura EL, Bijovsy AT. The cytostome of *Trypanosoma cruzi* epimastigotes is associated with the flagellar complex. *Exp Parasitol.* 1999; 92(4): 223-31.

[43]   Porto-Carreiro I, Attias MA, Miranda K, de Souza W, Cunha-e-Silva N. *Trypanosoma cruzi* epimastigote endocytic pathway: cargo enters the cytostome and passes through an early endosomal network before storage in reservosomos. *Eur J Cell Biol.* 2000; 70: 858–69.

[44]   Soares MJ. The Reservosome of Trypanosoma cruzi epimastigotes: an organelle of the endocytic pathway with a role on metacyclogenesis. *Mem Inst Oswaldo Cruz, Rio de Janeiro,* 1999; 94 (I): 139-41.

[45]   Cunha-e-Silva N, Sant'Anna C, Pereira MG, Porto-Carreiro I, Jeovanio AL, de Souza W. Reservosomes: multipurpose organelles? *Parasitol Res.* 2006; 99(4):325-7.

[46]   Docampo R, Jimenez V, King-Keller S, Li ZH, Moreno SN. The role of acidocalcisomes in the stress response of *Trypanosoma cruzi. Adv Parasitol.* 2011; 75: 307-24.

[47]   Kornberg A, Rao NN, Ault-Riche D. Inorganic polyphosphate: a molecule of many functions. *Annu Rev Biochem.* 1999; 68: 89–125.

[48]   Moreno SN, Docampo R. The role of acidocalcisomes in parasitic protists. *J Eukaryot Microbiol.* 2009; 56(3): 208-13.

[49]   Rohloff P, Montalvetti A, Docampo R. Acidocalcisomes and the contractile vacuole complex are involved in osmoregulation in *Trypanosoma cruzi. J Biol Chem.* 2004; 279: 52270–81.

[50]   Maugeri DA, Cannata JJ, Cazzulo JJ. *Glucose metabolism Essays Biochem.* 2011; 51: 15-30.

[51]   Bakker BM, Mensonides FI, Teusink B, van Hoek P, Michels PA, Westerhoff HV. Compartmentation protects trypanosomes from the

dangerous design of glycolysis. *Proc Natl Acad Sci U S A. 2000*; 97(5): 2087-92.

[52] Igoillo-Esteve M, Maugeri D, Stern AL, Beluardi P, Cazzulo JJ. The pentose   phosphate   pathway in *Trypanosoma   cruzi*: a potential target for the chemotherapy of Chagas disease. *An Acad Bras Cienc*. 2007; 79(4): 649-63.

[53] Parodi-Talice A, Durán R, Arrambide N, Prieto V, Piñeyro MD, Pritsch O, Cayota A, Cerveñansky C, Robello C. Proteome analysis of the causative agent of Chagas disease: Trypan*osoma cruzi. Int J Parasitol*. 2004; 34(8): 881-6.

[54] Martínez-Calvillo S, Vizuet-de-Rueda JC, Florencio-Martínez LE, Manning-Cela RG, Figueroa-Angulo EE. Gene expression in trypanosomatid parasites. *J Biomed Biotechnol*. 2010; 2010: 525241.

[55] Lima FM, Oliveira P, Mortara RA, Silveira JF, Bahia D. The challenge of Chagas' disease: has the human pathogen, *Trypanosoma cruzi*, learned how to modulate signaling events to subvert host cells? *N Biotechnol*. 2010; 27(6): 837-43.

[56] ElSayed NM, Myler PJ, Bartholomeu DC, Nilsson D, Aggarwal G, Tran AN,   Ghedin E, Worthey EA, Delcher AL, Blandin G, Westenberger SJ, Caler E, Cerqueira GC, Branche C, Haas B, Anupama A, Arner E, Aslund L, Attipoe P, Bontempi E, Bringaud F, Burton P, Cadag E, Campbell DA, Carrington M, Crabtree J, Darban H, da Silveira JF, de Jong P, Edwards K, Englund PT, Fazelina G, Feldblyum T, Ferella M, Frasch AC, Gull K, Horn D, Hou L, Huang Y, Kindlund E, Klingbeil M,Kluge S, Koo H, Lacerda D, Levin MJ, Lorenzi H, Louie T, Machado CR, McCulloch R, McKenna A, Mizuno Y, Mottram JC, Nelson S, Ochaya S, Osoegawa K, PaiG, Parsons M, Pentony M, Pettersson U, Pop M, Ramirez JL, Rinta J, Robertson L, Salzberg SL, Sanchez DO, Seyler A, Sharma R, Shetty J, Simpson AJ, Sisk E,Tammi MT, Tarleton R, Teixeira S, Van Aken S, Vogt C, Ward PN, Wickstead B, Wortman J, White O, Fraser CM, Stuart KD, Andersson B. The genome sequence of Tryp*anosoma cruzi*, etiologic agent of Chagas disease. *Science*. 2005; 309(5733): 409-15.

[57] Fernandes MP, Inada NM, Chiaratti MR, Araújo FF, Meirelles FV, Correia MT, Coelho LC, Alves MJ, Gadelha FR, Vercesi AE. Mechanism of *Trypanosoma cruzi* death induced by *Cratylia mollis* seed lectin. *J Bioenerg Biomembr*. 2010; 42(1): 69-78.

[58] Cadenas E. Mitochondrial free radical production and cell signaling. *Mol Aspects Med*. 2004; 25(1-2): 17-26.

[59] Lukes J, Hashimi H, Zíková A. Unexplained complexity of the mitochondrial genome and transcriptome in kinetoplastid flagellates. *Curr Genet.* 2005; 48(5): 277-99.

[60] Alves CR, Albuquerque-Cunha JM, Mello CB, Garcia ES, Nogueira NF, Bourguingnon SC, de Souza W, Azambuja P, Gonzalez MS. *Trypanosoma cruzi*: attachment to perimicrovillar membrane glycoproteins of Rhodnius prolixus. *Exp Parasitol.* 2007; 116(1): 44-52.

[61] Ciccarelli A, Araujo L, Batlle A, Lombardo E. Effect of haemin on growth, protein content and the antioxidant defence system in *Trypanosoma cruzi. Parasitology.* 2007; 134(Pt 7): 959-65.

[62] Moreno SN, Silva J, Vercesi AE, Docampo R. Cytosolic-free calcium elevation in *T. cruzi* is requeired for cell invasion. *J Exp Med.* 1994; 180(4): 1535-40.

[63] Fernandes MC, Andrews NW. Host cell invasion by *Trypanosoma cruzi*: a unique strategy that promotes persistence. *FEMS* 2012; 36(3): 734-47.

[64] Torrecilhas AC, Schumacher RI, Alves MJ, Colli W.Vesicles as carriers of virulence factors in parasitic protozoan diseases. *Microbes Infect.* 2012; 14(15): 1465-74.

In: Chagas Disease   ISBN: 978-1-62808-681-2
Editors: F. R. Gadelha, E.d.F. Peloso   © 2013 Nova Science Publishers, Inc.

Chapter III

Epidemiology of Chagas Disease

João Carlos Pinto Dias[1] and José Rodrigues Coura[2]

[1]Medicine (Tropical Medicine)
Emerit Researcher of the Oswaldo Cruz Foundation
Oswaldo Cruz Foundation, Belo Horizonte, Brazil
[2]Medicine (Infections and Parasitics Diseases)
Emerit Researcher of the Oswaldo Cruz Foundation
Oswaldo Cruz Foundation, Belo Horizonte, Brazil

Abstract

A brief revision of the epidemiology of American Trypanosomiasis is presented, emphasizing the most relevant and practical aspects related to Human Chagas Disease (HCD). Existing for 10 thousand years, and discovered in 1909 by Carlos Chagas, HCD was originally restricted to the American Continent, with an epidemiological summit in the twentieth eentury (incidence, prevalence and morbidity). Following the implementation of control programs and the intensification of the socio-economic urban and industrial model, the incidence of HCD was reduced, parallel with human cases spreading to urban spaces and non-endemic regions, and changes occurring in the disease profile of morbidity. Some predictable epidemiological risks and perspectives are considered at the end of this chapter.

Introduction

Chagas Disease (American Trypanosomiasis) was originally an enzootic disease, involving wild mammals and reduviidae insects. The natural history of its etiological agent, the protozoan *Trypanosoma cruzi* (*T. cruzi*) started about 80 million years ago, occurring in different sylvan sceneries of the tropical and subtropical American Continent. This primitive cycle began when hematophagous insects (*Hemiptera, Reduviidae, Triatominae*), derived from ancient Hemiptera (predators and phytophagous), were dispersed by America during the Upper Cretaceous. Later on it became a typical zoonosis (or antropo-zoonosis) affecting human beings and domestic and synanthropic mammals, in the so-called domestic cycle. Humans arrived in the Americas between 20,000 and 12,000 years ago, initially as nomads living by hunting. Small settlements appeared in rural areas, linked to an incipient agriculture and the domestication of animals (rabbits, guinea pigs, llamas, etc.). Primitive houses and abundant blood meal attracted native triatomine bugs. The parasite was brought into domestic areas by these insects, by wild reservoirs and domesticated animals, such as rabbits and guinea pigs ("cuyes") [1-7].

Detected in human mummies who lived in Latin America at least 4 million of years ago in focal and restricted social clusters, HCD was progressively being spread as an endemic disease, deeply related to socioeconomic parameters (mining and agricultural exploitation, migration, living standards) and bio-ecological situations (natural landscape, altitude, environmental temperature, humidity and other variables related to the vectors and reservoirs) [2, 3, 8-11]. The major expansion of HCD started with the European conquest of the New Word, depending basically on the political, economic and social scenery of Latin American (LA) colonization. For centuries, the disease was restricted to rural settlements, with a socio-political context strongly marked by very weak macro policies of production [12-14]. Undoubtedly, the summit of HCD endemicity occurred in the first half of the twentieth century, when the rural population of LA was very high and just before the implementation of regular vector and blood control programs in some countries. Since then, the tendency of a model urban-industrial spread throughout the Continent, also contributed to the reduction of vector transmission in Latin America [15]. The geographical distribution of American Trypanosomiasis extends continentally, from the Southern United States to Southern Argentina and Chile. It is currently estimated that more than 45 million human beings are exposed to the infection in this region, with a prevalence of about 8 million infected individuals [16]. In the last century, the globalization phenomena influenced important changes in LA, including national and international emigration of infected individuals, increasing the risk of HCD transmitted by blood transfusion, organ transplantation and congenital routes, in urban spaces of endemic and non endemic countries [5]. In the whole layout of American Trypanosomiasis, domestic and sylvan cycles of the parasite are integrated in a very dynamic and complex relation. The principal routes for *T. cruzi* transmission in the wild cycle are vectorial and oral, the last one involving the ingestion of contaminated vectors or reservoirs by susceptible mammals. Vectors have been mainly responsible for HCD transmission, followed by blood transfusion and congenital routes. The infection is generally benign in the enzootic cycle, in contrast with human disease, in which morbidity and mortality are significant and regional patterns of evolution exist. Given its characteristic originally enzootic, involving dozens of native species of vectors and reservoirs, the eradication of American Trypanosomiasis must be considered to be impossible. Nevertheless, considering particularly HCD, its control is perfectly plausible, by fighting regularly against the vectors domiciled, epidemiological surveillance, selection of donors in blood banks and adequate medical attention to already infected individuals [17, 18].

In this chapter we present a practical view of the epidemiology of HCD is intended, in the framework of present scenarios and of its principal expectations for the next decades.

Some Epidemiological Considerations about the Parasite

Since 1964, *T.cruzi* was classified in the *Stercoraria* group of trypanosomes, subgenus *Schizotrypanum* [11, 19]. Different populations of the parasite exhibit marked morphological, immunological, drug sensitivity and pathogenic diversity, depending on the host and other as yet undetermined factors, as well as regional and individual different clinical patterns of HCD and experimental infection. Recently, an international scientific consensus established the existence of at least six major groups of the "*T. cruzi* complex", accordingly to several biochemical, genetic and molecular parameters, distributed in different regions of America. In this distribution, probably different species of the vector (acting as a filter to select determined populations of the parasite) are involved, an epidemiological fact strictly dependent on the geographical landscape and of anthropic actions [1, 3, 7, 20]. The differentiation of epimastigotes into metacyclic trypomastigotes is influenced by the species of the vector, by the temperature and possibly by situations related to the insect (stress and some feeding components), being crucial in terms of the parasite transmission [11]. Once in the mammalian host, the parasite is able to invade different tissues and organs, causing cell destruction, inflammatory responses, fibrosis etc. The most important clinical consequences in HCD concern tissue damage at the level of the heart, the esophagus, the colon and the nervous system. Different populations of the parasite have different pathogenic impact in the host, in terms of morbidity, mortality and organ/tissue localization [10, 21].

The Vectors of American Trypanosomiasis

Triatomines are hemimetabolic insects, most of them spread in different American ecosystems. Although a few species can be eventually detected in other continents such as Asia, Africa and Australia, the natural *T. cruzi* infection of vectors and vertebrate hosts was never described outside of America [1, 5, 9, 22]. About 140 triatomine species have been found to be potential *T. cruzi* vectors, the majority being associated with birds, in sylvan ecotopes. A tentative systematization of the species is found in Table 1.

The principal transmitter species by region are: *Triatoma infestans, Pantrongylus megistus, T. brasiliensis, T. pseudomaculata, T. maculata, T. sordida, Rhodnius neglectus* and *R. nasutus* (South America), *R. prolixus, T. dimidiata* and *R. ecuadoriensis* (Andean Region), *R. prolixus* and *Triatoma dimidiata* (Central America) and *Phyllosoma* complex (Mexico). In the Panamá and Amazon Region, individuals of the genus *Rhodnius* (*R. pallescens, R. pictipes, R. brethesi*, etc.) do not colonize human dwellings, but the adults are able to invade them and eventually transmit the parasite [4, 10, 22, 25]. The dispersion of triatomines can be active (they have very limited capacity to walk and fly), or passive (eggs and nymphs transported by birds, by human movements (travelling, changes of residence, fire wood collection from wild environments, etc.) [20, 22, 24, 25].

The life cycle of the triatomines is completed in one or two years, according the species and general environment conditions, mainly temperature and humidity [1, 10, 22]. There are five larval instars from the egg to the adult stage, all of them able to get and to transmit the parasite [3, 22].

Table 1. Tentative classification of triatomines, according to their bio ecological characteristics and capacity of domestication [23, 24]

Group	Main characteristics of the species	Main Species	Observations
1	Strong adaptation to artificial ecotopes	*Triatoma infestans, T. rubrofasciata, Rhodnius prolixus*	Rare or non-existent wild foci
2	In the process of adapting to domestic situations, but still very present in wild foci *	*T.dimidiata, T. sordida, T. maculata, T. brasiliensis, T. pseudomaculata, T. barberi, T. longipenis, Panstrongylus megistus.*	Very dynamic between intra and peridomicile
3	Predominantly wild, with occasional forays into artificial ecotopes.	*Triatoma rubrovaria, T. protracta, Triatoma tibiamaculata, T. vitticeps, T. matogrossensis, R. neglectus, R. nasutus, R. pictipes, R. robustus, R. pallescens. R.ecuadoriensis.*	Exceptionally, adult insects can be detected in human dwellings, where rarely small colonies occur.
4	Essentially wild.	*T. arthurneivai, T. platensis, P.geniculatus, P. lutzi, P. diasi, R. robustus, R. pallescens*	Very occasional forays into artificial ecotopes, where small colonies rarely can be established
5	Exclusively wild	*Psammolestes sp., Cavernicola sp., Dipetalogaster maximus, Microtriatoma sp., Belminus sp.*	

* In the case of some species such as *P. megistus* and *T. dimidiata*, there are places (in Bahia, Brazil, and some Central America regions, respectively) where their adaptation to artificial ecotopes is almost complete, in spite of existing eventual foci in wild environment.

Strictly hematophagous, the insect needs at least one blood meal to change each stage of evolution [25, 26].

Several biologic and ethologic characteristics of each species have epidemiological significance in terms of HCD transmission, being the most important the capacity to colonize human dwellings, mainly indoors [20, 22, 25]. In this sense, *T. infestans* and *R. prolixus* have the higher capacity of colonization, being able to form intradomestic colonies of 1,000 individuals or more. In contrast, *Psammolestes tertius*, inhabiting exclusively in bird nests, never invades artificial ecotopes, while other species, highly dispersed around human settlements, such as *T. rubrovaria*, rarely invade and colonize indoor spaces. *P. megistus, T. dimidiata* and *T. brasiliensis* are native species with high capacity to invade and colonize human habitats. Once indoors, the density (number of insects per house) and the proportion of infected triatomines are considered epidemiologically very important. Regarding their feeding preferences, the great majority of triatomines are ornitophylic, but some prefer human blood (*T. infestans*). Some houses can be concomitantly infested by two species that generally occupy different spaces. In the case of T. infestans and T. sordida, the last prefers to live in henhouses, while the former remains associated with human beings [1, 22, 24, 26]. Considering the transmission of the parasite, those species with less time between the ingestion of blood and defecation are considered more efficient. For instance, the interval meal-defecation of *T. vitticeps* is too long (15-30 minutes), in contrast with *R. prolixus*, a very competent vector, with a time of 1-5 minutes. In terms of longevity and survival, triatomines basically require food and shelter. So, epidemiologically, very poor mud huts, overpopulated and filled with cracks and other hiding places are much more appropriate to HCD transmission than clean and hygienic masonry houses. All the triatomines are susceptible to *T. cruzi* infection, but the parasite is not pathogenic to them. The insect acquires the infection by sucking an infected reservoir, in any of its evolution stage. Once infected, they remain positive for the rest of their life. Notwithstanding, some laboratory observations show situations of a decrease on the parasite density, or even its virtual elimination, in longitudinal studies [3, 9, 22, 25]. Vertical transmission of *T. cruzi* do not exists amongst triatomines, but transmission by means of coprophagy and cannibalism is possible and has been described in experimental models [22, 25, 27, 28]. Also, the adaptation existing between the strain of the parasite and the local/regional triatomines species is important, since regional populations of T. cruzi are much more adapted to the vectors of the same region. This epidemiological fact is used to explain the clinical homogeneity of HCD in different geographic spaces [3, 4, 8, 10]. Vector control has been considered the principal tool to face HCD, since the 1940´s when Emmanuel Dias and other researchers employed the first effective long action insecticides against domestic triatomines and developed the strategy for a massive Public Health campaign [4, 15]. With regular and continuous action, almost strictly carried out by national and regional control programs, vector populations of the principal domestic species were being progressive and drastically reduced, especially those strictly domestic (*T. infestans* and *R. prolixus*) that were virtually eliminated in several regions [8, 15, 18]. Peridomestic and wild species are also vulnerable to the modern insecticides (Pyrethroids), but are more difficult to be controlled since multiple environmental conditions (light, wind, humidity, open and complex spaces, accessibility) hinder and make the chemical strategy less effective [4, 10, 17, 22]. The resistance of triatomines to the commonly employed insecticides is possible and was registered in the past with chlorine products (*R. prolixus* in Venezuela) and in recent years with pyrethroid compounds (*T. infestans*) in areas of Bolivia and Argentina [4, 6, 22]. This is a preoccupant subject, to be monitored and driven by governmental institutions, in strict participation with the WHO [4, 17, 18]. Fortunately, the episodes described until now (and several laboratory trials) revealed that the triatomines resistance is restricted to determined family of insecticides (chlorine, pyrethroids), being vulnerable to others (carbamates, organophosphate) [15, 26].

The Mammal Reservoirs of *T.cruzi*

For its evolution, the parasite demands one stage in the insect (vector) and the other in superior vertebrates, considered as its natural reservoirs. About 100, or more, wild reservoirs of *T. cruzi* have been described, all of them pertaining to the class *mammalia*. In general, small or medium mammals are more susceptible.. Animal hosts in endemic area include rodents, bats, dogs, cats, rabbits, opossums, racoons and armadillos. The transmission of *T. cruzi* amongst non-human reservoirs can be accomplished mainly by means of vector and oral routes, according to the circumstances. For instance, monkeys and marsupials used to eat triatomines, while dogs and cats eat several species of rats, which can be infected [1, 27, 29]. Of particular importance are the so-called *synanthropic* reservoirs, which live in sylvan environments but commonly move to human proximity, making a bridge between the wild enzootic and the domestic cycles. This is the case of different marsupial and wild rats, plentiful dispersed along the endemic area. There are a wide variety of infection rates in the natural hosts of *T. cruzi*, being the parasitaemia usually higher in young and newly infected animals. In general, the natural infection is benign in wild reservoirs but, on the experimental side, acute disease, cardiopathy and digestive "megas" can be obtained in dogs, mice and small rodents [3, 10, 27]. Another remarkable fact with possible epidemiological significance is the existence of a double cycle of the parasite in the same host,

Didelphis sp., one of them being the classical systemic cycle and the other restricted to the anal glands of the animal, both being able to produce infective *T. cruzi* forms [4, 30].

The Importance of Birds and Other Vertebrates Not Susceptible to *T. cruzi* Infection

Other non-mammal vertebrates are involved in the ecology of American Trypanosomiasis, being important food source for triatomines, especially at the sylvatic and peridomestic environments. Birds have also an additional role in triatomine hosting and dispersion, by giving them shelter through their nests and by carrying nymphs and eggs in plumage, sometimes for long distances [1, 3, 22].

Mechanisms of Parasite Transmission

They can be divided in two groups: a) the main mechanisms, by means of vectors (triatomines), blood transfusion, oral transmission (contaminated food) and congenital transmission (placental or birth canal) and, b) the secondary mechanisms, involving organ transplantation, laboratory accidents (management of vectors, reservoirs, cultures of the parasite etc.), sexual route (contact with contaminated sperm or menstrual fluid) and, hypothetically, deliberate criminal contamination [4, 31]. Some principal aspects of the epidemiology of HCD transmission can be summarized as follows [3, 8, 10, 26, 32, 33].

Vectorial transmission: it is responsible for more than 70% of the existing cases of HCD, with antecedents having lived in rural infested areas of endemic countries. It occurs when metacyclic trypomastigote forms of *T. cruzi* found in the dejections of infected triatomines penetrate actively in the vertebrate host through the intact mucosa or a solution of continuity in the skin. In the environment, parasites will remain alive and viable for some time (minutes) after the dejection, depending on chemical and physical factors, particularly the temperature (ideal between 20 and 30ºC), pH (around 7.2) and humidity (ideal above 80%) [9, 10, 27]. In reality, this kind of transmission does not happen easily, since it depends on several factors such as the vector density, the number of contaminative contacts, the proportion of infected insects, the size of the inoculum, possible defenses in the site of penetration, etc. [3, 11].

In the majority of the cases HCD is transmitted indoors in human dwellings highly colonized by infected triatomines, generally during the night and in hot weather. Nevertheless, peridomestic transmission can occur when people have the custom of sleeping outside, in regions of extreme heat, e.g. [22, 28]. As a general rule, the incidence of HCD is drastically reduced in areas under vector control and/or housing improvement. For instance, the prevalence of *T. cruzi* infection among scholar children of Bambui, Brazil (an hyperendemic municipality with more than 75% of rural dwellings infested by *T. infestans*) was 46% in 1948, when acute cases of HCD were frequent. Once regular vector control was installed (1955) acute cases disappeared and the childhood infection prevalence decreased to 11% in the 1960´s, to 3% in 1974 and to 0% in the 1980´s, remaining negative until today [34]. The same was observed in other well-controlled areas, such as in Uruguay, São Paulo State (Brazil) and in some Provinces of Argentina and Chile, where acute cases disappeared and the prevalence of the infection in children, pregnant women and blood donors was reduced progressively [16, 18, 28].

Transfusion transmitted HCD: the risk of its occurrence for a single 500 ml bottle of total blood elicited from an infected (chronic) donor varies from 12 to 25%, but can be higher in hyper endemic regions [23, 35]. The incidence of transfusion transmission in the absence of adequate blood control will depend basically on the prevalence of infected donors in the region, on the number of transfusions received by the susceptible individual and on the parasitemic level of the donors. The transmission can occur by means of the transfusion of total blood, plasma and other blood components (red blood cells concentrate, cryoglobuline, platelets concentrate etc.), remaining infective as the parasite stoked in refrigerated material up to 15 days [35]. Besides the progressive control of blood banks in most of the endemic countries, a cohort effect has been observed when vector control was implemented, showing a drastic reduction in the proportion of infected donors, mainly in low age groups [3, 36, 37]. As an example, in Brazil, the general prevalence of infected donors in 1991 was higher than 2.0%, decreasing to 0.21% in 2005. The global prevalence of infected blood donors along Latin America varies from 0.4% (Brazil) to more than 20% (certain Bolivian regions), being calculated at a general rate of 2.47% for the region, in 2006 [16].

Congenital Chagas Disease: In 2006, there was an estimated 14,385 congenital cases of HCD per year in Latin America plus the USA, with an incidence rate of 0.133 cases per every 100 babies born, varying from 0.573 in Bolivia to 0.039 in Uruguay. The total number of infected women in the fertile age (15-44 years) was calculated in 1,809,507 [16]. Similar to what happens with infected blood donors, a progressive reduction of infected pregnant women has been observed in Brazil and Uruguay as a result of vector control, mainly in low age groups, indicating that in one or two decades, cases of congenital transmission of HCD will be an exception [34]. Congenital transmission may occur at any time during the pregnancy, being more probable in the last six months, generally involving the colonization of the placenta by the parasite. The risk of congenital transmission is higher in the pregnant human presenting acute disease or higher parasitemia in the chronic phase [3, 19, 38]. The morbidity of congenital HCD is usually low: the majority of the babies are born asymptomatic, only a small portion (less than 10%) present severe states of immaturity, low birth weight, cardiopathy, mega oesophagus or meningoencephalitis [38]. Once it is presently impossible to prevent congenital transmission among infected pregnant women, the best procedure is the detection of serologic positive pregnant women and the immediate treatment of the infected babies. As it is not always possible to detect the parasite in new born individuals and because they have circulating antibodies (IgG delivered from the infected mother) until the age of 6-7 months, the basic strategy to face the asymptomatic congenital HCD consists of the execution of a conventional serology around the 8-9 months of the babies life, treating specifically those who present positive results [10, 23, 29, 39].

Oral transmitted Chagas Disease: It is usual in the enzootic cycle and can be reproduced easily in several experimental situations. In terms of HCD, the event is virtually unpredictable, but the majority of the registered cases occurred during hot season, in rural or peri-urban spaces, in a vicinity with wild vegetation or other natural and artificial ecotopes able to shelter triatomines and mammal hosts of the parasite [4, 40]. Familiar and group outbreaks have been detected since the decade of the 1970's in Brazil, involving the ingestion of contaminated food such as rice, soups, milk and different juices (sugar cane, açai, guacaba guayaba). Not always exceptional, but not yet registered, could be the occurrence of oral transmission in the context of hunters and primitive ethnical groups who have the tradition to eat crude meat of wild animals (armadillos, opossums, rodents) or even triatomine bugs [29, 41]. The source of the parasite is usually related to the presence of infected triatomines around the cooking place, but possible ingestion of reservoir meat and marsupial secretions also have been supposed [1, 4, 10, 29]. The first detected outbreak occurred in Teutônia, Rio Grande do Sul State (Brazil), affecting concomitantly more than 20 individuals, probably due to a traditional meal (rice, beans, meat) probably contaminated by opossum dejection. Later other cases appeared in Belém and Pará States (Brazil), supposedly by soup contaminated with triatomines (or their dejections). Other important outbreaks were detected in Paraiba and Santa Catarina States (Brazil) (due to contaminated sugar cane), followed by the detection of several outbreaks likely caused by oral transmission in the Amazon Region (Brazil), accumulating about 400 cases until today [4, 42]. In other countries, oral transmission was also detected in Venezuela, Colombia, Mexico and Ecuador [4]. The parasite can remain alive and infective up to two weeks or more, in different kinds of food & juices not submitted to high temperatures. The penetration in the host is accomplished by means of the mucosa, from the moth cavity until the duodenum. To overcome the stomach barrier (gastric acidity), the parasite covers itself with a capping of mucin-like glycoproteins [40, 43].

The accidental route: at least 100 cases are known by the *chagalogists*, generally involving technicians or researchers who deal with the parasite, vectors and reservoirs (including human cases). In research laboratories, accidents have been detected in eye contamination by triatomines dejections or blood drops blown from infected animals, as well as in accidental aspiration of liquid culture of the parasite, and even in cases of perforating injuries caused by surgical instruments during the manipulation of infected animal. More exceptional have been accidents by the aspiration of aerosol originated from centrifugation of infected materials [11, 29].

It is recommended that technicians be submitted to periodic serology, be trained to minimize the risk of infection in their activities, adequately employ the usual protection equipment to deal with infected materials and receive regular supervision of senior personnel. It is mandatory to start the specific treatment (during 10 days) immediately after a supposed contamination [3, 31, 32].

The transmission by organ transplantation: Since the 1980s, several cases were reported in different endemic (Argentina, Brazil, Venezuela, Chile) and non-endemic (USA, Spain, France) countries, involving infected donors and susceptible recipients. The majority of the cases were of kidney transplantation, but also were registered in the transmission of heart transplantation and, possibly, in bone marrow and pancreas transplantations [8, 31]. According to epidemiological antecedents, serology for Chagas Disease must be performed in donor and recipient, before the surgery. The necessary employment of immunosuppressive drugs, to minimize rejections of the recipient, used to increase the parasitemic level and the severity of acute HCD in the majority of the cases, imposing immediate diagnosis and specific treatment [29, 33].

When the transplant is imperative, if the donor is infected and not the recipient, the specific treatment of the donor during ten days before the surgery and of the recipient during at least ten days after the surgery can be indicated [29].

The other mentioned mechanisms are really of exception and lack of epidemiological importance. It remains to be said that the transmission through breast milk, often speculated in several texts or lectures, is basically a case of oral transmission. Its occurrence is quite exceptional, and should never serve as a reason to prohibit the breastfeeding, except in cases of a woman being in the acute phase or with bleeding on the nipples [26, 32].

Geographical Distribution Incidence and Prevalence of HCD

American Trypanosomiasis had its origin in the continental space extending from the Southern USA to Southern Argentina and Chile, where infected vectors, reservoirs and human beings have been found naturally infected by *T. cruzi*. The major prevalence of HCD correspond to those territories occupied by *T. infestans* and *R. prolixus*, followed by *T. dimidiata* and *T. brasiliensis*, just because these species have the major capacity to colonize human dwellings. In a general way, HCD occurs in those spaces ecologically defined as "open spaces", where human intervention deeply changed the natural environment, also offering their houses for vector and reservoir shelter [1, 20, 25].

Regional patterns of incidence and morbidity were precociously appointed by different authors, probably being related to variations involving different vectors and parasite populations [1, 3, 7, 44].

For an overview of HCD in the Americas the countries were divided into four groups, according to the vectors involved, the morbidity and the organization of transmission control (Table 2). Of course, important variations may occur within a country, as epidemiological patterns specific, being emblematic the situation in the Amazon, involving nine countries of South America. This table can be complemented by specific information about the distribution of the different groups of the parasite; in general, group II predominates in the south of the Amazon Region, being almost absent north of the equator. On the other hand, group 1, widely dispersed, characterizes the sylvatic cycle of Trypanosomiasis [4, 8, 22].

Table 2. Chagas Disease: Four groups of epidemiological patterns in endemic countries of Latin America and USA, in the beginning of the XXI Century (modified from [10])

Groups	Countries	Epidemiological characteristics	Observations
I	Argentina, Bolivia, Brazil, Chile, Ecuador, Honduras, Paraguay, Peru, Uruguay and Venezuela	Domestic cycles with areas of high prevalence of HCD. Predominance of chronic cardiopathy. Presence of digestive forms below Equator Line. Important sylvatic cycles in several different natural environments. Main vectors: *T. infestans, R.prolixus, T. brasiliensis, T. dimidiata, T. pseudomaculata, T.maculata, T. sordida.* Sylvatic foci of *T. infestans* in restricted areas of Bolivia and Chile.	Existing vectorial and transfusion control programs in the majority of the Countries. Perspective of elimination of *T. infestans and R.prolixus* in areas where these species are exclusively domestic.
II	Colombia, Costa Rica and Mexico	Detected domestic and sylvatic cycles. Transmission detected in blood banks. Presence of chronic cardiopathy. Main vectors: *T. dimidiata* and *Phyllosoma* complex	Vector control programs incipient or absent. Control of blood banks being improved.
III	El Salvador, Guatemala, Nicarágua and Panamá.	Detected domestic and sylvatic cycles. Transmission detected in blood banks. Scarce clinical information, with the detection of chronic cardiopathy and, eventually mega-. Main vectors: *T dimidiata, R.prolixus* (in extinction) and *R. pallescens* (Panamá)	Vector control programs existing in Guatemala and Nicaragua, partially in El Salvador.
IV	Antilhas, Bahamas, Belize, Cuba, USA, Guyanas, Haiti, Jamaica, Suriname.	Detected sylvatic cycle. Rare and scarce autoctonus cases of HCD. Little clinical information. No domestic triatomines. More than 300,000 chronic individuals living in USA, in total majority comprised of immigrants from Latin America.	Absence of control programs.

Concerning the incidence and prevalence of HCD in recent years, data estimated by PAHO [16] in 2006 are summarized in Table 3.

The scenarios and epidemiological parameters of HCD are dynamic and have undergone major changes, especially from the twentieth century. In particular, with the implementation of adequate vector and transfusion control (in parallel with human development, health education and epidemiological surveillance), the impact of HCD was significantly reduced in the last twenty years, as shown by Moncayo & Silveira in Table 4 [18].

Table 3. Rates of annual incidence by vector transmission* and prevalence** of HCD estimated for AL in coming years to 2005, according to PAHO [16]

Region/country	Incidence	Prevalence	Total of infected individuals
Southern Cone	0.005	1.714	4,451,900
Andean Countries	0.011	1.029	1,168,000
Central America & Belize	0.005	1.159	310,000
FR. Guayana, Guyana & Suriname	0.029	1.288	18,000
Mexico	0.007	1.028	1,100,000
Total (Latin America)	0.008	1.448	7,694,500

* New cases of vector transmission by 100 inhabitants.
** Number of infected individuals (any mechanism of transmission) per 100 inhabitants.

Table 4. Changes in epidemiological parameters of HCD in Southern Cone of Latin America, 1990-2006 according to WHO/TDR [18]*

Epidemiological parameters	1990	2000	2006
Annual deaths	(>) 45,000	21,000	12,500
Annual new cases	700,000	200,000	41,200
Prevalence (million cases)	30	18	15
Population at risk (million individuals)	100	40	28

Launching of a Regional Control Initiative in 1991, with vector and blood bank control being highly strengthened in seven Countries. HCD transmission considered interrupted in Uruguay (1987), Chile (1999) and Brazil (2006), later on being certified in some areas in Argentina, Paraguay and Bolivia [16].

Pragmatically, for epidemiological purposes, serological screenings in non-selected populations are very useful to determine the prevalence and the incidence of HCD. For classical endemic areas, curves presenting high positivity in low age groups are revealing active transmission, in contrast with figures where positive cases appear only in higher age groups, meaning the transmission occurred many years ago (controlled areas).

To estimate incidence, serology performed in lower age groups is very useful, as well as the detection of new positive cases of previously negative individuals [3, 45].

The Case of Amazon

Considered for a long time as a non-endemic region for HCD, in recent decades the Amazon has called the attention of researchers and Public Health workers to more than 400 acute cases detected mainly in Pará State, Brazil. Most of them are related to *T. cruzi* 1, Z3 and hybrid Z1Z3 [4]. The Amazon was never was free of the presence of *T. cruzi*, since an intense enzootic cycle is spread all over the region, involving about 25 species of the vector (mainly of the *Rhodnius* gender, frequently infected by the parasite) and a great diversity of wild *T. cruzi* hosts (marsupials, bats, rodents, edentates, carnivores, primates etc.) [41]. In the particular region of Barcellos, Amazonas State, Brazil, a very particular situation involves active vector transmission of HCD, by means of *R. brethesi,* a triatomine living in *piaçaba* palm tree, that attacks people who work collecting leaves and fibers of this tree, used in the regional broom industry [41]. Between 1988 and 2005, Pinto et al. [42] studied 233 acute cases of Brazilian Amazon, most of them in the States of Pará and Amapá: 78.5% of these cases were probably transmitted by the oral route, by means of familial outbreaks (affecting a mean of 4 individuals/outbreak), with a mortality of 5.6% (in majority due to acute myocarditis). All of the cases were autoctonous, most were adults, detected mainly between August and December. No domiciliated triatomines were found, but reports of adult insects invading houses are frequent in the region [41, 46]. The possibility of passive introduction of alien species carried by human immigration from endemic areas (*T. infestans, T. brasiliensis, P. megistus, T. dimidiata* etc) in the Amazon was suggested in the past but fortunately, was never detected [29, 46]. Acute cases have also been detected in the Amazon Region of other countries such as Ecuador, Colombia and Venezuela [41, 46]. Nevertheless, the chronic form of HCD is considered to present low endemicity in the Amazon, measured by a low prevalence among blood donors and proportional mortality well below the national average in Brazil [26, 46]. Even so, severe isolated cases can be found among autoctonous individuals, basically corresponding to chronic heart disease [4]. Digestive chronic forms seem to be extremely rare in the region [46]. Today it is recognized that HCD in the Amazon occurs, in a very particular way, with a still low prevalence and morbidity of chronic disease, but with an apparent increase of acute cases resulting from the proximity of the enzootic cycle with human populations, making oral transmission possible and eventually, by means of triatomine invasion. This is an unpredictable situation, for which the basic prevention presumes to keep the houses distant to the forest, good practices in food hygiene and the epidemiological surveillance for suspected individuals, with prompt diagnosis and treatment of the cases and exploitation of their contacts. As the most frequent symptom of Amazonian acute cases is fever, malaria technicians are being trained, in Brazil, to identify *T. cruzi* in their routine microscopy [4, 42]. In summary, it seems to be true that HCD in the Amazon Region today constitutes a worrisome problem of Public Health, although not as serious as that which occurred in the classical endemic areas, which is much more difficult to prevent [4, 18, 41].

Chagas Disease in Non Endemic Countries

Out of the American Continent, triatomines can be found in small and very limited sylvatic or peri urban foci in Asia, Africa, and the Pacific Region, probably having spread via maritime trade from Latin America, as early as the sixteenth century [5]. *T. cruzi* has not been detected in such triatomines. The principal species found out of America is *Triatoma rubrofasciata*, generally associated with rats and one murine trypanosome, the *T. conorhini*, not pathogenic to human beings [29]. Natural *T. cruzi* infection of wild reservoirs also was never detected, suggesting the non-existence of the enzootic cycle outside the American Continent. On the other hand, *T. cruzi* has been spread from endemic to non-endemic countries by means of the progressive migration of infected individuals [4, 5]. Since the 1960s, a combination of economic hardships and political turmoil, the latter reinforced by economic stagnation, forced an increased migration from Latin America to North America, Europe, Australia and Asia [5, 13]. The proportion of migrants infected by *T. cruzi* depends on their origin, social status and age group, ranging from roughly between 2 and 5% [13]. It has been calculated that USA is the country that received the highest number of infected migrants (above 300,000), followed by Spain (86,711), the sum of other European countries (more than 7,000) and Australia (more than 3,000) [5, 13]. The origin of chagasic migrants to the USA is principally Mexico and Central America, while South American infected migrants were predominant in Spain, Canada and Australia, around 2006. To Japan, the migration of chagasic individuals was basically from Brazil and Peru [5, 13]. Historically, the intensity of the migration movement from endemic to non-endemic countries has changed in the last 30 years. From South America, 954,000 migrants in 1990, 1,702,465 in 2000, and 2,310,500 in 2006 were registered. The numbers for Central America and Mexico were 5,613,000, 11,155,725 and 14,378.672 respectively [13]. In recent years, however, resulting from the world social and economic crisis, these waves of migration are being changed; the migration to non endemic regions is being restrained, in parallel with a tendency to migrants going back to their countries of origin [14]. Once the infected individuals are installed in non-endemic regions, cases of transfusion, congenital transmission and by organ transplantation, in addition to cases of sudden death, of co-infection with HIV, etc., begin to be detected. Medical and social care to these individuals can be complicated, concerning with their legal situation in the new country, since in many cases these are clandestine people, without the right to attend regular medical services [14].

Finally, in the last years, several efforts have being made in non-endemic countries to face the disease and its consequences out of Latin America. Awareness that Chagas disease is now found in places far from endemic areas of Latin America is important because it leads to the development of strategies to prevent potential sources of transmission (e.g., blood transfusion, organ transplantation, or congenital transmission), and to identify individuals who may benefit from anti-parasitic therapy [5].

Morbidity and Mortality

There are epidemiological parameters, which vary greatly according to the region and the population ("regional nuances of DCH"). The acute form of infection is usually inapparent or oligosymptomatic, with an average mortality between 2% and 9%, always higher in those non-treated cases at lower ages and clinically more exuberant. Major vector pressure always results in higher intensity of transmission, mainly to younger individuals, in which acute disease is more severe [33]. Some data suggest that the morbidity and mortality in acute HCD are higher in black individuals [28]. In the chronic form, there are important regional differences; the incidence of digestive forms the north of the equator line being significantly lower, in comparison with the Central Brazil, for example. Regarding the chronic cardiopathy, it is more frequent and severe in Minas Gerais and Goiás States (Brazil) than in the other areas such as Rio Grande do Sul (Brazil) and Central America. For Brazil, as a whole, the incidence of chronic chagasic cardiopathy varies between 20 and 35% in adult individuals, and the digestive forms between 5 and 15% [23, 39]. The *mortality* is generally high among individuals who develop severe forms of chagasic heart disease, especially those resenting advanced cardiac failure and/or complexes and multiple arrhythmias. This means, roughly, that about

5% of Brazilian chagasic patients, at least, are doomed to die due to DCH, which corresponds to 100,000 individuals (considering the estimate prevalence of 2,000,000 chagasic people today existing in the Country. Considering the official registration of obits in Brazil the annual incidence of deaths due to HCD has varied between 5.4 and 4.1 per 100,000 inhabitants, that is, oscillating around 6,000 deaths/year, with a small tendency to decrease since the 1980´s [9, 16, 29]. Nevertheless, in micro regions of elevated endemicity, the mortality among infected adult individuals can be much higher. For instance, longitudinal studies among infected individuals presenting chronic heart Chagas in Minas Gerais and Bahia (Brazil), show that 60% of the deaths were due to HCD [26, 34]. In the acute phase, mortality occurs mainly among younger children, due to acute myocarditis and or meningoencephalitis. Death in chronic HCD is generally predominant in the male gender, in a proportion that varies between 1.5 to 2:1, particularly between 30 and 50 years of age, thus contributing significantly to the reduction of life expectancy in endemic areas [34]. The early deaths in DCH have high social significance, either directly (by a large number of years of productive life lost), or indirectly (by unimaginable costs to the orphans and the widows in families already poor, when the father (and provider) dies relatively young) [3, 8]. In general, the majority of the chagasic patients die of sudden death, primarily due to the cardiac tachyarrhythmias, but a large number also die of heart failure, frequently associated with thromboembolic situations. In the case of sudden deaths, the final mechanism is generally the ventricular fibrillation, a product of ventricular tachycardia, paroxysmal originated from arrhythmias extra-systolic frequent and complex [10, 29]. In the last three decades, with the improvement of therapeutic resources for cardiopathy management, a progressive increase of life expectancy has been observed in well assisted chagasic individuals, an epidemiological fact that reinforces the need of adequate medical and social attention in endemic and non-endemic areas [4, 23]. Regarding the digestive side, the basic (or unique) cause of death in HCD is the sigmoid volvulus, a complication relatively frequent in advanced megacolon that requires immediate and adequate medical intervention [28, 47, 48].

The Whole Society Facing Chagas Disease

Some social and institutional considerations about the control and the medical attention of HCD are also opportune. Considering the usual poverty of chagasic populations all over the world, the role of the State in coping with the disease is crucial [14, 17, 49]. Control programs have been executed by governmental agencies in Latin America, generally leaded by the Ministries of Health. Today, in the new model of decentralization of health activities, control and surveillance programs were allocated at the municipal levels, making the homogeneity, the coverage, and the sustainability of vector control very complicated [14, 17, 49]. Control of blood banks is easier to perform, basically depending on continuous supervision and quality control [12, 37]. Decentralized programs, when well established, should be able to reach prompt and effective epidemiological surveillance, since in the municipality are the houses, the vectors and the patients, and where political will can easily be influential. Nevertheless, program continuity, depending only on peripheral levels is not easy. Regional references for technical advice, laboratory help and continuous supervision are extremely opportune and necessary in decentralized systems. For instance, the situation of a vector program in Brazil is presently highly deficient, in terms of coverage and epidemiological information, since the federal level completely lost its technical capacity and because regional references (Health State Secretaries) – with few exceptions – did not effectively assume their role in the program [4, 14, 18, 49, 50]. In terms of medical attention, the main problems involve access, expertise and continuity. HCD is a typical health problem requiring different degrees of complexity in health care.

Most of the chronic infected patients are in the indeterminate form, basically requiring regular (annual) revisions by a general clinician, who eventually will indicate specific treatment. This is clearly possible for Primary Health decentralized systems, depending on a minimum organization, not yet installed in the great majority of municipalities [50]. Severe Chagas disease chronic cases will demand tertiary attention, meaning about 5 to 10% of the existing cases, that is, between 400 and 800 thousand cases, in majority very poor and dependent on the State [9, 14]. Nevertheless, an organized and regular system including more specialized references to HCD attention does not exist in endemic countries [50-52]. Finally, at the more optimistic side, it should be mentioned that two new and complementary elements have been engaged in the fight against HCD, both emerged from the scientific community engaged with the problem: the Intergovernmental Initiatives against Chagas Disease, launched in Southern Cone, 1991, and the progressive and highly beneficial adhesion of important NGOs (DNDI, MSF) in the global efforts to maintain sustainable actions and pertinent research. In addition, the definitive inclusion of Chagas Disease in the official agenda of WHO, since 2010, has been very opportune [5].

The Future

The epidemiological summit of HCD incidence and morbidity has happened in the middle of the twentieth century and was progressively overtaken by means of regular vector and blood bank control, in parallel with socio-political changes as urbanization and rural migration. Incidence, prevalence and morbidity were reduced in several endemic areas, some of them being declared free of transmission. Nevertheless, there is still much to do, to face this disease that still threatens around 28 million people. The predictable scenarios for HCD in the three next decades include the reduction of incidence, prevalence and morbidity, besides a residual situation of focal transmission in those poorest and more isolated endemic areas, or in those where control programs are not implemented, sustained or technically problematic. This is the case of poor residual counties in Northeast Brazil, the complicated ecological and political area of the Great Chaco, in South America, the complex ecologic situation of the Amazon Region and the political situation of Mexico, where a regular and continuous control program was never implemented for lack of political will [4, 15, 49, 50, 53]. And naturally, the major epidemiological tasks will be referred to the basic scenarios involving secondary species of triatomines, peridomestic environment, poverty and political decisions [4, 14, 15, 53].

Looking at the future, the main challenges regarding HCD as a Public Health problem may be considered as: 1) To consolidate vector and blood bank control in Latin American countries still without regular control programs; 2) To implement regular and sustainable epidemiological surveillance in those countries with advanced control programs; 3) To detect and to give medical and social attention to around 12-14 million of yet uninfected people both in endemic and non-endemic countries. By the way, the present and future scenarios involve a progressive reduction of disease visibility and the need for permanent surveillance regarding savage triatomines and possibly new epidemiological situations. The basic strategy in this task was basically the research and the publication of epidemiological data, pointing out the medical and social frame of the disease, in terms of its geographical distribution, incidence, prevalence, morbidity, mortality and social costs. In the last three decades, it has been recognized that the social and economic aspects of HCD were extremely important in the production and in the dispersion of the disease. Moreover, this "contextual" frame was shown to be clearly linked with the clinical aspects, also being determinant in the possibilities of disease control and management. The definitive fight against HCD cannot be focused simply in the traditional biological angle, but must involve all those aspects and determinants of its occurrence, *"understanding the "chagasic" patient in his bio-psycho-social and cultural reality, in a political and economic context in which the common denominator is poverty"* [53].

Some predictable risks involving Chagas Disease for the next two decades [4, 17, 49, 50, 53]

Epidemiological:
Recrudescence of classical vectors = LOW
Increasing of housing colonization by wild vectors = LOW
Appearance of new endemic areas of vector transmission= LOW
Recrudescence of transmission in blood banks = VERY LOW
Increase of congenital transmission = VERY LOW
Increase of oral transmission = unpredictable

Institutional:
Difficulties in decentralized structures = HIGH
Loss of interest and reduction of resources at the government level, in endemic countries = MEDIUM/HIGH
Decrease of priority in PAHO and WHO = possible
Loss of consistency & effectiveness of the current Intergovernmental Initiatives = POSSIBLE

Scientific:
Lack of priority and financial help = HIGH
Decreasing scientific interest = MEDIUM/HIGH

Political:
Major decrease of priority = HIGH

Final Considerations

Until now, the main effective social impulse to face Chagas Disease has come from the Scientific Community engaged with the problem all around the world. Since Carlos Chagas and Emmanuel Dias, several years ago, scientists have making extraordinary efforts to initiate and sustain the fight against the disease, constantly advocating the cause of HCD victims to politicians and governors. Although somewhat successful, such efforts must be maintained for at least two or three decades more, according to the epidemiological situation [4, 13, 14, 17]. In such a perspective, a tentative scoring of the main risks involving the future of HCD is presented, as a way to finish this small chapter with some provocative questions regarding the epidemiology of the American Trypanosomiasis.

References

[1] Barretto MP. Epidemiologia. In Brener Z, Andrade ZA (Orgs) Trypanosoma cruzi e Doença de Chagas, Rio de Janeiro, Guanabara Koogan ED. 1979; 89-151.

[2] Araújo A, Jansen AM, Reinhard K, Ferreira LF. Paleoparasitology of Chagas disease. A review. *Mem Inst Oswaldo Cruz.* 2009; 104 (Suppl. 1): 9-16.

[3] Dias JCP, Coura JR. Epidemiologia. In Dias JCP and Coura JR (orgs) Clínica e Terapêutica da doença de Chagas. Uma abordagem para o clínico geral. Fiocruz Ed., Rio de Janeiro. 1997; 33-66.

[4] Coura JR, Dias JCP. Epidemiology, control and surveillance of Chagas disease – 100 years after its Discovery. *Mem Inst Oswaldo Cruz.* 2009; 104: 31-40.

[5] Coura JR, Albajar-Viñas P. Chagas disease: a new worldwide challenge. *Nature Outlook.* 2010; S6-S7.

[6] World Health Organization. Control of Chagas Disease. Second report of a WHO expert committee. *Technical Report Series Nr. 905, Geneva.* 2002.

[7] Zingales B, Andrade SG, Briones MRS, Campbell DA, Chiari E, Fernandes O, Guhl F, Lages-Silva E, Macedo AM, Machado CR, Miles MA, Romanha AJ, Sturm NR, Tibayrenc M, Schijman A. A new consensus for Trypanosoma cruzi intraspecific nomenclature: second

revision meeting recommends TcI to TcVI. *Mem Inst Oswaldo Cruz.* 2009; 107: 1051-54.

[8]   Miles MA, Yeo M, Gaunt MW. Epidemiology of American Trypanosomiasis. In: Maudlin I, Holmes PH, Miles MA (orgs.) *The Trypanosomes.* London. CABI Publishing. 2004; 243-51.

[9]   Antunes CMF. The epidemiology of Chagas disease. In Gilles HM (orgs) Protozooal Diseases. Arnold, London. 1999; Chapt 4, 351-69.

[10] Carlier Y, Dias JCP, Luquetti AO, Honteberye M, Torrico F, Truyens C. Trypanosomiase Américaine ou maladie de Chagas. *Encyclopedie Medico- Chirurgicale.* (Maladies infectieuses). Elsevier, Paris. 2002; 8-505-A-20.

[11] Brener Z. Trypanosoma cruzi: morfologia e ciclo evolutivo. In Dias JCP and Coura JR. (orgs) Clínica e Terapêutica da doença de Chagas. *Uma abordagem para o clínico geral.* Fiocruz Ed., Rio de Janeiro. 1997; 25-32.

[12] Schmunis GA. Enfermedad de Chagas en un mundo global. In OPS & Fundación Mundo Sano. La enfermedad de Chagas a la puerta de los 100 años del conocimiento de una endemia americana ancestral. Washington: Publ. OPS/CD/426-06. 2007; 251-66.

[13] Schmunis GA. Chagas diease in Latin America and its dissemination to the developed world. *Rev Soc Bras Med Trop* 2009; 42: 29-35.

[14] Dias JCP, Coura JR. Globalizaton and Chagas Disease. In Delic Z (organ.) *Globalization and responsibility.* Rijeka (Croatia), InTech Ed. 2012; 153-66.

[15] Dias JCP, Schofield CJ. The evolution of Chagas disease (American Trypanosomiasis) control after 90 years since Carlos Chagas discovery. *Mem Inst Oswaldo Cruz.* 1999; 94: 103-22.

[16] Organización Panamericana de La Salud. Estimación cuantitativa de la enfermedad de Chagas en las Americas. Documento OPS/HDM/CD/425-06. Washington. 2006; 28.

[17] Dias JCP, Silveira AC, Schofield CJ. The impact of Chagas Disease in Latin America; a review. *Mem Inst Oswaldo Cruz.* 2002; 97: 603-12.

[18] Moncayo A, Silveira AC. Current epidemiological trends for Chagas disease in Latin America and future challenges in epidemiology, surveillance health policy. *Mem Inst Oswaldo Cruz.* 2009; 104: 17-30.

[19] Hoare C. *The Trypanosomes of mammals. A zoological monograph.* Blackwell scientific Publication, Oxford-Edinburg. 1972; 749.

[20] Forattini OP. Biogeografia, origem e distribuição da domiciliação de triatomíneos no Brasil. *Rev Saud Publ* 1980; 15: 265-99.

[21] Andrade LO, Machado CR, Chiari E, Pena SD, Macedo AM. Differential tissue distribution of diverse clones of Trypanosoma cruzi in infected mice. *Mol. Biochem Parasitol* 1999; 100: 163-72.

[22] Schofield CJ. Triatominae: Biologia y Control. *Eurocommunica* Publications. London. 1994.

[23] Ferreira MS, Lopes ER, Chapadeiro E, Dias JCP, Luquetti AO. Doença de Chaga. In Veronesi R and Foccacia R (orgs) Tratado de Infectologia. São Paulo, Atheneu Ed. 1996; 1175-1213.

[24] Lent H, Wigodzinsky P. Revision of the Triatominae (Hemiptera, Reduviidae) and their significance as vectors of Chagas' disease. *Bull Am Mus Nat History.* 1979; 163: 125-250.

[25] Sherlock I. Vetores. In Brener Z, Andrade ZA and Barral Neto M. Trypanosoma cruzi e doença de Chagas (II. Ed.), Rio de Janeiro: Guanabara Koogan. 2000; 21-40.

[26] Dias JCP. Epidemiologia. In Brener Z, Andrade, ZA and Barral-Neto M (orgs.). Trypanosoma. cruzi e doença de Chagas (II Ed.), Rio de Janeiro, Guanabara Koogan Edit. 2000; 48-74.

[27] Dias E. Estudos sobre o Schizotrypanum cruzi. *Mem Inst Oswaldo Cruz.* 1934; 1-326.

[28] Dias JCP, Silveira AC, Schofield CJ. The impact of Chagas Disease in Latin America; a review. *Mem Inst Oswaldo Cruz.* 2002; 97: 603-12.

[29] Dias JCP, Macedo VO. Doença de Chagas In: Coura JR. *Dinâmica das Doenças Infecciosas e Parasitárias.* Rio de Janeiro, Guanabara Koogan. 2005; 557-93.

[30] Deane MP, Lenzi HL, Jansen A. Trypanosoma cruzi: vertebrate and invertebrate cycles in the same mammal host, the opossum Didelphis marsupialis. *Mem Inst Oswaldo Cruz.* 1984; 79: 513-15.

[31] Dias JCP. Mecanismos de transmissão. In Brener Z, Andrade ZA and Barral Neto M. *Trypanosoma cruzi e doença de Chagas* (2a. Edição), Rio de Janeiro: Guanabara Koogan. 1979; 152-74.

[32] Amato Neto V, Lopes MH, Umezawa ES, Ruocco RMSA, Dias JCP. Outras formas de transmissão do Trypanosoma cruzi. *Rev Patol Trop.* 2000; 29: 115-29.

[33] Dias JCP, Amato Neto V, Luna EJA. Mecanismos alternativos de transmissão do Tripanonoma cruzi no Brasil e sugestões para sua prevenção. *Rev Soc Bras Med Trop* 2011; 44: 375-379.

[34] Dias JCP. Longitudinal studies on human Chagas disease in Bambuí, Minas Gerais, Brazil. *Rev Soc Bras Med Trop.* 2009; 42: 61-8.

[35] Cerisola JA, Rabinovich A, Alvarez M, Corleto A, Pruneda J. *Enfermedad de Chagas y la transfusion de sangre.* Bol of Sanit Panam 1972; 73: 203-21.

[36] Wendel S. Doença de Chagas transfusional. In Dias JCP and Coura JR (eds), Clínica e Terapêutica da Doença de Chagas. *Um Manual Prático para o Clínico Geral,* Fiocruz, Rio de Janeiro. 1997; 411-28.

[37] Moraes-Sousa H, Ferreira-Silva MM. Control of transfusion transmission of Chagas disease in different Brazilian regions. *Rev Soc Bras Med Trop.* 2009; 42: 103-05.

[38] Moya P, Moretti ERA. Doença de Chagas Congênita. In Dias JCP and Coura JR. (orgs) Clínica e Terapêutica da doença de Chagas. *Uma abordagem para o clínico geral.* Fiocruz Ed., Rio de Janeiro. 1997; 383-410.

[39] Secretaria de Vigilância em Saúde do Ministério da Saúde. Consenso Brasileiro em Doença de Chagas. *Rev Soc Bras Med Trop.* 2005; 38: 29.

[40] Dias JCP. Notas sobre o Trypanosoma cruzi e suas características bio-ecológicas, como agente de enfermidades transmitidas por alimentos. *Rev Soc Bras Med Trop.* 2006; 39: 370-75.

[41] Aguilar HM, Abad-Franch F, Dias JCP, Junqueira ACV, Coura JR. Chagas disease in the Amazon Region. *Mem Inst Oswaldo Cruz.* 2007; 102: 47-55.

[42] Pinto AYN, Valente SA, Ferreira Jr AG, Coura JR. Fase aguda da doença de Chagas na Amazônia Brasileira. Estudo de 233 casos do Pará, Amapá e Maranhão, observados entre 1988 e 2005. *Rev Soc Bras Med Trop.* 2008; 41: 602-14.

[43] Buscaglia CA, Campo VA, Frash CA, Noia JMD. Trypanosoma cruzi surface mucins: host dependent coat diversity. *Nature Rev Microbiol.* 2006; 4: 229-36.

[44] Laranja FS, Dias E, Nóbrega GC, Miranda A. Chagas' disease. A clinical, epidemiologic and pathologic study. *Circulation.* 1956; 14: 1035-60.

[45] Luquetti AO, Castro AM. Diagnóstico sorológico da doença de Chagas. In Dias JCP and Coura JR. (orgs) *Clínica e Terapêutica da doença de Chagas. Uma abordagem para o clínico geral.* Fiocruz Ed., Rio de Janeiro. 1997; 9-114.

[46] Dias JCP, Prata A, Schofield CJ. Doença de Chagas na Amazônia: esboço da situação atual e perspectivas de prevenção. *Rev Soc Bras Med Trop.* 2002; 35: 669-78.

[47] Coura JR. Síntese histórica sobre a evolução dos conhecimentos sobre a doença de Chagas. In Dias JCP and Coura JR (orgs) Clínica e Terapêutica da doença de Chagas. *Uma abordagem para o clínico geral.* Fiocruz Ed., Rio de Janeiro. 1997; 469-86.

[48] Rezende JM, Moreira H. Forma digestiva da doença de Chagas. In: Brener Z, Andrade ZA and Barral Neto M. Trypanosoma cruzi e doença de Chagas. Rio de Janeiro: Guanabara Koogan. 2000; 297-343.

[49] Briceño-León R. La enfermedad de Chagas y las transformaciones sociales en America Latina. In OPS (organ.) La enfermedad de Chagas a la puerta del conocimiento de una endemia americana ancestral. OPS/CD/426-06, Washington. 2007; 219-30.

[50] Dias JCP. *Doença de Chagas, ambiente,* participação e Estado. *Cad Saude Publ* 2001; 17: 165-69.

[51] Dias JCP. Freqüência e importância das formas clínicas da doença de Chagas no Brasil. *Rev Soc Bras Med Trop.* 1996; 29: 103-05.

[52] Dias JCP. Atención del paciente infectado por el Trypanosoma cruzi en el sistema de salud: aspectos operativos y laborales. *Rev Patol Trop.* 1998; 27:159-75.

[53] Dias JCP, Briceño-León R, Storino R. Aspectos sociales, económicos, políticos y culturales. In: Storino,R. and Milei, J. (organ.) *Enfermedad de Chagas.* Doyma Argentina Ed., Buenos Aires. 1994; 527-48.

In: Chagas Disease   ISBN: 978-1-62808-681-2
Editors: F. R. Gadelha, E.d.F. Peloso   © 2013 Nova Science Publishers, Inc.

Chapter IV

Clinical Aspects of the Disease

Eros Antonio de Almeida
Universidade Estadual de Campinas,
Campinas-SP, Brazil

Abstract

Chagas disease is an endemic anthropozoonosis in Latin America caused by the flagellate protozoan *Trypanosoma cruzi* and transmitted to humans and other mammals by hematophagous triatomine bugs, which is the most significant mode of transmission in terms of public health. This disease has acute and chronic stages and various clinical forms. The symptomatology is polymorphic and depends on the stage and clinical form of the disease. In the acute stage, this disease behaves as an infectious disease that includes a point of entry leading to fever, malaise, asthenia, anorexia, headache, lymphadenopathy and hepato-splenomegaly. Meningoencephalitis and myocarditis sometimes can occur in younger children; these conditions are associated with the severe forms of the acute stage and can lead to death. Most patients in the chronic stage in endemic regions do not present with any symptomatology or changes in complementary exams and these patients are considered to have the undetermined form of the disease. The disease can progress to cardiopathy, which includes (in order of frequency) arrhythmias, blockages of the electrical stimulus conduction system, ventricular dysfunction and pulmonary and systemic thromboembolic events. Patients may experience palpitations, syncope and heart failure. The digestive system also can be affected, with dysphagia and constipation as the most frequent symptoms secondary to megaesophagus and megacolon. The treatment is palliative and nonspecific and is directed according to the clinical manifestations, as with other cardiopathies and digestive diseases. Specific treatment is directed to the parasite.

Introduction

Chagas disease or American trypanosomiasis is an endemic anthropozoonosis in Latin America caused by the flagellate protozoan *T. cruzi* and transmitted to humans and other mammals by hematophagous triatomine bugs [1]. Vectorial form and blood transfusion are the most significant forms of transmission from a public health standpoint. An acute stage follows infection; the chronic stage occurs approximately four months after infection. The chronic stage has a variable evolution in different clinical forms [1], some of which are associated with high morbidity and mortality. It is estimated that in Brazil, 1.8 to 2.4 million people are at this stage of the disease, with one third of them in the heart or digestive form[2]. Although expressive numbers are known, specific and effective therapy has not been achieved yet for *T. cruzi*. The available medications, benznidazole and nifurtimox, have low efficacy in the acute stage of the disease and may have serious side effects, such as digestive symptoms, peripheral neuropathy and allergic dermopathy, among others [3. In the chronic stage, such medications have shown questionable efficacy [4].

The acute stage of the disease has become increasingly rare in countries that are in control of blood and vector transmission, especially of the main bug, *Triatoma infestans* [5]. This change, as well as the social transformations generated by the process of urbanization in Latin America, has determined epidemiological changes in relation to Chagas disease. Patients in the chronic stage have begun to have longer survival times, which has led to the existence of comorbidities with clinical manifestations that overlap with those of Chagas disease and make diagnosis difficult.

The clinical manifestation is polymorphic, depends on the stage of the disease and is almost the same for all forms of parasite transmission. Thus, for a better understanding, the clinical features should be discussed according to the acute stage and the different forms of the chronic stage of Chagas disease.

Clinical Aspects of the Acute Stage of Chagas Disease

In the acute stage, Chagas disease behaves like parasitosis and is similar to infectious diseases in general. The symptoms/signs and the associated exams are closely related to those caused by the parasite *T. cruzi*, which must be present in the peripheral blood; the symptoms cease as the parasite disappears, and the patient is considered to be in the chronic stage. The acute stage described by Carlos Chagas [6] was confirmed by other observers, and no significant changes have been made to the description in the 100 years that followed the discovery of the disease. The acute stage begins up to 15 days after infection and lasts for approximately eight weeks. At this point, the signs of transmission, general clinical features and systemic abnormalities should be considered. The frequency and intensity can vary widely and are most likely related to the intensity of the parasitemia, which can generate clinical manifestations that go unnoticed along with other severe problems that may lead to death. Fortunately, most patients belong to the first group, where the clinical manifestation is nonspecific and does not lead to a diagnosis.

The point of entry of the parasite into the human body is essential for the diagnosis of the acute stage of Chagas disease, which involves complex ophthalmic-ganglionic manifestations (Romaña's sign) and inoculation chagoma. The first one consists of an asymmetrical bieyelid swelling with a rosy-violet color (Figure 1).

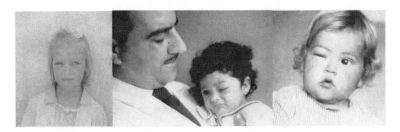

Figure 1. Oftalmoganglionar complex (Romaña's signal) in acute Chagas' disease.

The remarkable features that differentiate this condition from another etiology of eyelid edema are the absence of pain, the long duration that can take two months to completely disappear and the low level of conjunctival secretions. This condition is usually followed by conjunctival hyperemia, lymphonodomegaly and dissemination to the affected hemiface. The presence of dacryoadenitis is less frequent. Although Carlos Chagas had made reference to facial edema [6], he did not emphasize the diagnostic value that this sign would have for the acute stage of the disease, and diagnosis has become easier after this recognition. The frequency of this sign varies according to the observations of Argentinean authors [7], but it was found in approximately 50% of the cases that occurred in endemic regions.

The inoculation chagoma is the second most important point of entry of the parasite. This condition is an injury to the skin on any part of the body, but most often in those areas usually uncovered while sleeping. The lesion has a variable size and appears as an erythematous maculonodular lesion, but it may resemble a painless or slightly painful boil, almost never with suppuration. This latter feature is important in the differentiation from other infectious etiologies, particularly bacterial infections. The resolution of inoculation chagoma is also much longer than bacterial infections and occurs with satellite lymphonodomegaly. Other forms of the chagoma presentation are the hematogenous metastasis and lipochagoma of the cheek that occur in more severe cases [7]. In all cases, these signs are assumed to be closely related to the parasite, which is found in biopsies of these regions. Exceptions are made in some cases of Romaña's sign, which may be due to an allergic reaction to the parasite particles.

Fever stands out among the symptoms and general signs, and it appears in nearly all cases. However, the presentation of the fever is nonspecific and may be confused with other common causes, particularly in children during the first year of life. The fever can be remittent or intermittent with varying degrees of intensity, disappearing into lysis. The fever is remarkable for its greater intensity in the afternoon and prolonged duration, which may last for months. Other symptoms, such as malaise, asthenia, anorexia and headache, may be present concurrently. Although it should be considered as a general manifestation, edema has been highlighted as highly suggestive of this stage of trypanosomiasis. The edema is not related to the point of entry of the parasite and differs from the swelling observed in cases of heart or renal failure. This condition is generalized, elastic, without temperature variations, and is characterized by the absence of a positive godet sign. The pathogenesis is not well understood, but it occurs in more severe cases in small children.

The systemic changes that are usually found in infectious processes consist of lymphadenopathy; this condition is almost always present, affects various regions and is not associated with inflammatory signs. Hepatomegaly and splenomegaly are frequent, vary in size and are not associated with significant structural modifications. Exanthematous reactions, such as urticaria, morbilliform lesions or erythema polymorphe, also may occur.

More severe systemic changes, although less frequently observed, are those related to the heart and central nervous system. The clinical manifestation of cardiac involvement is acute myocarditis, which can be observed in other infectious diseases. There is no specific manifestation related to Chagas disease. Thus, it is important to observe the point of entry of the parasite, the general manifestations and the suggestive clinical features of the acute heart disease. The severity is variable, and the symptoms are most evident in more severe cases. Tachycardia is a frequent sign, but it is not related to fever. Hypophonesis of the heartbeat can be present, as well as mitral valve murmur or in the mesocardial region of low intensity as observed in functional murmurs. These findings may be part of the clinical manifestation of heart failure and can occur in varying degrees of severity. This condition can lead to patient death, and the specific treatment for *T. cruzi* beyond the usual treatment for heart failure is critical for a better prognosis [7]. Further examinations include those commonly used for morpho-functional cardiac evaluation, but these exams do not reveal specific changes. The electrocardiogram that has diagnostic value for Chagas disease in the chronic phase shows only sinus tachycardia, low QRS voltage, primary changes in ventricular repolarization and first degree atrioventricular block, which are entirely nonspecific changes.

The nervous form of the acute stage of Chagas disease is more severe, is responsible for patient death and occurs as acute meningoencephalitis. In this stage, seizures that are difficult to control may occur. Paralysis,motor incoordination, and behavioral disorders have also been observed. Less obvious symptoms can be found in lesser degrees of severity, such as irritability, continuous crying in younger children, headache, myalgia and insomnia. These symptoms are important, as they can draw attention to the diagnosis of acute Chagas disease in endemic areas. A cerebrospinal fluid examination can indicate meningitis along with biochemical and cellular nonspecific changes, and finding *T. cruzi* is essential for diagnosis. However, when *T. cruzi* is not detected, the diagnosis is not excluded if there is still clinical suspicion. In Chagas disease, the parasite is usually found in the cerebrospinal fluid examination after reactivation in the central nervous system in immunosuppressed patients [8]. This finding generally does not occur with the same frequency in the acute stage [7]. Severe forms of chagasic meningoencephalitis occur mostly in young children, infants and immunosuppressed. In the absence of a specific treatment against *T. cruzi,* the patient will eventually die. In areas where the vectorial transmission of Chagas disease has been controlled, meningoencephalitis can be found in immunosuppressed individuals, especially in those with AIDS, and the course of the disease is similar to that of the acute phase observed in endemic regions [9].

In general, the organism responds to the acute stage of Chagas disease systemically, and there may be symptomatology in all regions of the body. Persistent diarrhea, nausea and vomiting can occur in the digestive system, while bronchitis may be present in the respiratory system. Anemia, orchiepididymitis and mumps have also been described [7]. Complementary examinations, such as hemograms and measurements of erythrocyte sedimentation, C-reactive protein, protein electrophoresis, liver function and others, may show nonspecific changes that are common to other acute infectious diseases. Acute Chagas disease affects mainly young children but can occur at any stage of life. When nonspecific symptoms of acute infectious disease (especially fever) occur in individuals from endemic regions, Chagas disease should be considered among differential diagnoses. The clinical course is usually benign and disappears spontaneously. Less than 10% of cases show severe forms of myocarditis and meningoencephalitis, which may cause death. Furthermore, early diagnosis and specific treatment may change the poor prognosis of severe forms.

Clinical Aspects of the Chronic Stage of Chagas Disease

The clinical aspects of the chronic stage of Chagas disease are polymorphic and are related to the forms of the disease. After the conclusion of the acute phase, patients become asymptomatic in almost all cases without any manifestation of the disease for a period that can vary from approximately 20 years to a lifetime. At this time, the diagnosis of Chagas disease is only possible if serological tests or indirect parasitological evaluations are positive. Given the evolving character of Chagas disease, these asymptomatic patients are designated as having an indeterminate form and could present a defined clinical picture. As criteria for this classification, patients must be asymptomatic, test normal on a 12-lead electrocardiogram at rest, and have normal contrast radiographs of the esophagus and colon [10]. Individuals who progress to cardiac and digestive forms are those with clinical features defined as Chagas disease.

Chronic chagasic cardiopathy is manifested clinically by symptoms related to arrhythmias, conduction disturbances in the electrical stimulus, ventricular dysfunction and thromboembolic events that are either isolated or associated. At this point, the disease is not different from chronic cardiopathies of other etiologies; however, because it is a chronic fibrosing myocarditis, this condition has clinical features that vary widely in intensity, occur at a greater frequency, are severe and are difficult to control. Furthermore, this condition is associated with a high mortality rate [11].

The prevalent symptoms in chronic chagasic cardiopathy are closely linked to cardiac arrhythmias. The ventricular premature beat is the most common arrhythmia and, depending on the stage and severity of the disease. It can be found isolated and monomorphic or poliomorphics and acoplated (Figure 2).

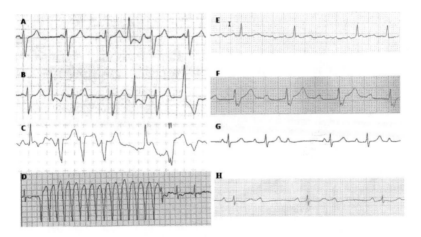

Figure 2. Eletrocardiogram: Arrhythmias in the chronic chagasic cardiopathy. A. Isolated ventricular premature beat; B. Frequent and complex ventricular premature beat; C. Non-sustained ventricular taquycardia; D. Sustained ventricular taquycardia; E. Atrial fibrillation; F. First degree atrioventricular block; G. Second degree atrioventricular block (Wenkebach); H. Total atrioventricular block.

The symptom reported by the patient is usually palpitation, or the feeling of the heartbeat, often called dropped beats. Such an alteration, without any ventricular dysfunction, does not require treatment unless the symptom is uncomfortable to the patient. Clinical examination by electrocardiogram, Holter and echocardiography should be repeated periodically to monitor the arrhythmia and the appearance of ventricular dysfunction. If treatment is necessary, the drug of choice should be amiodarone [11]. When arrhythmia gives rise to low cardiac output, symptoms such as presyncope and syncope are associated with the palpitations. The intensity of low cardiac output is highly variable, from simple palpitation to seizures (Stoks-Adams syndrome), and can occur alone or in combination. The crises start and stop suddenly, lasting minutes or hours, and occur with or without paleness, cold sweats, nausea, vomiting, weakness and chest pain as if it was myocardial ischemia. The arrhythmias responsible for such symptoms are usually sustained or non-sustained ventricular tachycardias (Figure 2) that are frequent in chronic chagasic cardiopathy. These arrhythmias far exceed other etiologies and lead to an arrhythmogenic cardiopathy. Such complex arrhythmias are responsible for the high morbidity and mortality observed in chronic chagasic cardiopathy because the patient dies when the arrhythmias degenerate into ventricular fibrillation [12]. Although not frequently, such arrhythmias can occur without any other symptoms, especially those observed in a 24-hour Holter measurement [13]. The electrocardiogram examination is necessary for a chagasic patient, regardless of symptoms, because this test can diagnose the cardiopathy [10]. In the presence of the symptoms reported as indicators of arrhythmias, two new tests have become essential as part of a good medical practice in the evaluation of these patients: Holter monitoring and echocardiography. The monitoring of cardiac rhythm for 24 hours can detect all types of arrhythmias in most cases of chronic cardiopathy. This exam directs the treatment, which can reverse symptoms and prevent death. If a Holter measurement is not possible, the conventional stress test has similar indications but with less sensitivity [14]. However, such testing does not always detect arrhythmias that justify the symptoms. In these situations, further invasive methods, such as programmed electrical stimulation, are necessary to reproduce the arrhythmia and occasionally to perform an ablation. Unfortunately, this type of treatment is less successful in chronic chagasic cardiopathy than in other etiologies, possibly because chronic chagasic cardiopathy is a progressive fibrosing myocarditis. Other tests used in the investigation of cardiopathy, such as myocardial scintillography, cardiac catheterization, magnetic resonance and others, can assist in the differentiation of Chagas disease from other etiologies and may eventually be used in the investigation of arrhythmias in chronic chagasic cardiopathy.

The prognosis of arrhythmias in chronic chagasic cardiopathy is linked to the presence of ventricular dysfunction, similar to the cardiopathies of other etiologies. However, in chronic chagasic cardiopathy, complex arrhythmias may occur with the risk of death even in the absence of or in mild ventricular dysfunction, which is uncommon [13]. Thus, echocardiography constitutes an essential supplementary test in the evaluation of individuals with chronic chagasic cardiopathy, regardless of symptoms [10], but mainly those with symptoms suggestive of arrhythmia. In these situations, the treatment of arrhythmias is formally indicated, either by medication or by electrical cardioversion. The latter is mostly used for sustained ventricular tachycardia with hemodynamic alterations; this method can obtain a rapid and effective reversal of symptoms, is well tolerated by patients and should be followed by pharmacological treatment. Antiarrhythmics of all classes have been used in the treatment of arrhythmias in chronic chagasic cardiopathy, but the best results were found using amiodarone [15]. This drug is a class III antiarrhythmic associated with few serious adverse effects in doses of 600 mg daily for 10 days to start treatment and 200 to 400 mg daily for maintenance. Although amiodarone can cause sinus bradycardia and blockages in the conduction of cardiac electrical stimulation, its use is not contraindicated in chronic chagasic cardiopathy. Branch and fascicular blockages occur frequently with this cardiopathy, but they rarely worsen during treatment. However, prolonging the QT interval can cause a proarrhythmic effect with an induction of polymorphic ventricular tachycardia (*torsade de pointes*). In patients using amiodarone, it is necessary to routinely monitor thyroid function, ocular and pulmonary deposition, hyperpigmentation of the skin, and changes in digestive and neurological function. In general, these adverse effects depend on the dose and period of use, and dose reduction or discontinuation of treatment maybe necessary depending on the intensity or nature of the event. Among these extracardiac effects, the most severe is the deposition in the lung parenchyma resulting in pneumonitis and fibrosis; fortunately, these adverse events are rarely observed with the doses used in Brazil. The treatment should be discontinued once this change is detected [16]. Options to treatment with amiodarone have been propafenone, mexiletine and sotalol. The non-pharmacological options are catheter or surgical ablation and implantable cardioverter-defibrillators for cases of refractory ventricular tachyarrhythmias [15]. Atrial fibrillation comprises another type of cardiac arrhythmia that can induce symptoms in chronic chagasic cardiopathy (Figure 2). However, atrial fibrillation is not frequent and is generally observed in the later stages of cardiopathy, and contributing to a bad prognosis [17]. The diagnosis is confirmed by conventional electrocardiogram, and the treatment does not differ from that for atrial fibrillation. Treatment focuses on the reduction of heart rate, restoration of the sinus rhythm and prevention of thromboembolic events, and the strategies usually employed for these purposes are similar to the ones used for other cardiopathies.

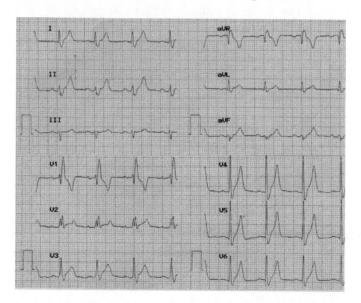

Figure 3. Chronic chagasic cardiopathy. Eletrocardiogram with left anterior fascicular block and right bundle branch block.

The clinical aspects described for tachyarrhythmias in chronic chagasic cardiopathy can be the same as observed in patients with bradyarrhythmias. In this cardiopathy, the occurrence of atrioventricular blockages and sinus node disease is common, and these symptoms appear at all levels of severity. Thus, syncope is the most striking symptom resulting from this type of bradycardia, especially when associated with the third-degree atrioventricular block (Figure 2). The bradyarrhythmia diagnosis is performed using the same methods described above for tachyarrhythmias, stressing the importance of conventional and dynamic electrocardiograms. The electrophysiological exams verify the locations where atrioventricular blockage occurs, which reflects the clinical picture, prognosis and treatment [16]. In chronic chagasic cardiopathy, the blockage is more severe because it is usually below the atrioventricular node. The same applies for the study of the sinoatrial node, especially when medications such as amiodarone and beta-adrenergic blockers are used, which may aggravate possible node disease. The treatment of bradyarrhythmias consists of the implantation of a cardiac artificial pacemaker, and it has been documented that this action benefits the patient by controlling symptoms, improving quality of life and increasing survival [15]. Concomitant bradyarrhythmias and tachyarrhythmias are common in chronic chagasic cardiopathy; therefore, treatment for both situations may be necessary for a complete remission of symptoms and to improve survival.

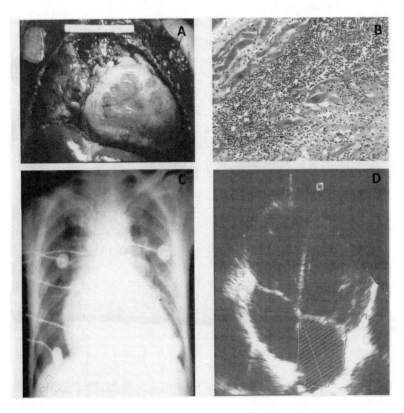

Figure 4. Anatomopatological, radiographical and ecocardiografical aspects of the chronic chagasic cardiopathy. A. Autopsy - Severe global cardiomegalia; B. Chronic miocardite and fibrose; C. Thorax X-ray - Severe global cardiomegalia and pulmonary congestion; C. Ecocardiogram - Severe global dilatation.

A clinical aspect that corresponds to the trademark of chronic chagasic cardiopathy is the high incidence of sudden death, which has close ties with the frequency of the severe arrhythmias described above. These cardiac abnormalities are the principal cause of death in chronic chagasic cardiopathy (accounting for two thirds of deaths), especially in the earlier stages of the disease. Even more serious is the fact that unexpectedly sudden death can occur in patients with mild ventricular dysfunction or in the absence of any dysfunction [18]. The pathogenic mechanisms of chronic chagasic cardiopathy, including inflammation, fibrosis, conduction disturbances of electrical stimulation of the heart and neurovegetative disorders, support the severity of this cardiopathy, including sudden death.

The most common disturbances in the conduction of electrical cardiac stimulation found in chronic chagasic cardiopathy are blockages of the right bundle branch and the anterior fascicle of the left branch (Figure 3). The combination of these two blockages can be considered as a diagnosis of chronic chagasic cardiopathy in individuals from endemic regions due to the high frequency with which it is found [19]. Such intraventricular blockages are asymptomatic but can be detected by electrocardiogram, stressing the value of this test for the diagnosis of chronic chagasic cardiopathy.

Another relevant clinical aspect is heart failure that meets the advanced stages of chronic chagasic cardiopathy. This condition is associated with poor prognosis due to a higher mortality than heart failure secondary to other etiologies [20]. This type of heart failure is congestive with a predominant systolic deficit (Figure 4).

Although ventricular dysfunction is bilateral, the initial symptom is a progressive dyspnea with exertion, indicating failure of the left ventricle. Next, there is edema of the lower limbs, and the classic symptoms of congestive syndrome emerge with disease progression. Anasarca and cavity effusions occur, which involve the right ventricle. After right ventricular dysfunction is established, the clinical signs of pulmonary congestion become less prominent. Thus, the reported symptoms and results of the physical examination should be valued for detection of early stages of myocardial dysfunction. Echocardiography has a special value because it is able to identify systolic dysfunction and structural changes of the heart before the onset of heart failure can be detected by clinical examination, which enables the early introduction of therapeutic measures [10]. Usually, all the clinical signs described here are present in decompensated chronic chagasic cardiopathy. Thus, in addition to echocardiography, all the other exams listed above are warranted at this stage of the disease. As for heart failure secondary to other heart diseases, treatment should be based on the use of diuretics, angiotensin-converting enzyme inhibitors or specific receptors and beta adrenergic blockers, and should be optimized according to the individual [16, 21]. Because there are no long-term placebo-controlled prospective studies involving the drugs currently used to treat heart failure in patients with chronic chagasic cardiopathy, the entire treatment is based on studies of heart failure from other etiologies. Thus, in the absence of contraindications, spironolactone, hydralazine, nitrates and digitalis can be added in doses and periods commonly used in other cardiopathies. Given the severity, higher doses may be required, such as for diuretics, as the congestive systemic aspect is predominant. Other medications are typically required, such as antiarrhythmics and anticoagulants; however, use of these drugs concurrently with other treatment may cause drug interactions. In addition, antiarrhythmics, digitalis and beta blockers are bradycardic, which can accentuate the bradycardia naturally found in chronic chagasic cardiopathy as a result of blockages and sinoatrial node dysfunction. Cardiac transplantation is an alternative for individuals in the final stages of the cardiopathy, in which medical treatment is not sufficient to control the disease [15]. Parasitic disease without specific effective treatment is not a formal contraindication for transplantation. A specific treatment, with benznidazole has been effective in controlling a reactivation of Chagas disease and the clinical progression of transplant patients has been similar or better than in non-chagasic individuals. However, organs from donors with Chagas disease have not been used, according to standards of the Brazilian legislation, given the potential possibility of transmitting Chagas disease [15].

Thromboembolic events are often described in chronic chagasic cardiopathy [20]. These events are mainly related to the presence of heart failure. However, mural thrombosis in the cardiac chambers is frequent regardless of ventricular dysfunction, which makes this disease unique in terms of thromboembolic events. One of the peculiarities of this cardiopathy is the presence of apical lesions on the left ventricle, a marker of Chagas disease, which is the origin of thrombosis in almost 100% of cases observed in autopsies (Figure 5).

However, thrombi are found in all cardiac chambers, with both systemic and pulmonary embolisms occurring. The arrhythmias described above are part of the thrombogenic potential of chronic chagasic cardiopathy and, therefore, enabling a higher incidence of embolisms. The emboli of the lungs and brain are more clinically relevant, and chagasic cardiopathy is an independent risk factor for stroke in endemic regions [20]. Thus, anticoagulation therapy should be part of the therapeutic treatment of chronic chagasic cardiopathy, using warfarin, antiplatelets or heparin, especially when there is heart failure, detection of intracavitary thrombus or potentially thrombogenic arrhythmias, such as atrial fibrillation. The monitoring of complications of anticoagulation should be performed in compliance with the standard contraindications.

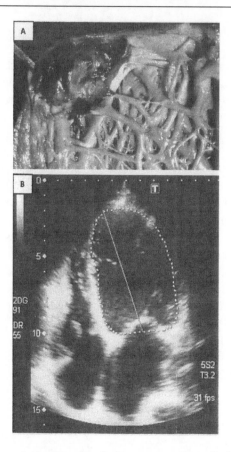

Figure 5. Chronic chagasic cardiopathy. A. Anatomopatology - Left ventricle with apical aneurysm and thrombus; B. Ecocardiogram - Left ventricle with apical aneurysm.

Although the cardiac form is the most frequent and severe clinical manifestation of chronic Chagas disease, approximately 20% of individuals experience problems with the digestive system, particularly the esophagus and colon [21]. The clinical aspects are due to damage of the intrinsic nervous system of the digestive tube (the myenteric plexus of Auerbach) by the inflammation resulting from parasite and host-parasite interactions that generates neuronal destruction and motor dysfunction of the loops. The denervation occurs throughout the digestive tube, irregularly and in a variable intensity, but the esophagus and terminal colon are the most frequent sites of clinical manifestation. At the end stage of this disease, these segments are typically dilated, resulting in megaesophagus and megacolon (Figure 6);

however, the symptoms and diagnosis of the impairment of the loops may occur before this stage.

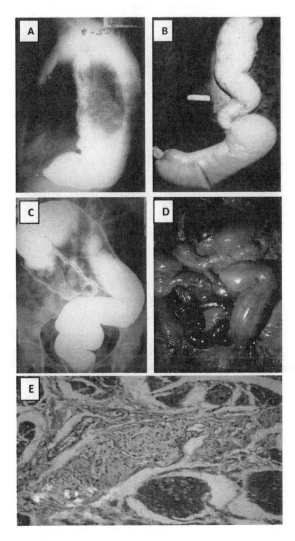

Figure 6. Anatomopathological and radiographical illustration of megaesophagus and megacolon. A. Esophagogram - Megaesophagus degree IV; B. Anatomical image with severe megaesophagus; C. Colon X-ray with megacolon; D. Anatomical image with dilatation of sigmoid segment; E. Ganglionite of plexus intramural of the intestine with absence of neurons.

The impairment of the digestive tube manifested as megaesophagus or megacolon can occur in isolation or can be associated with heart disease. In addition, these impairments vary widely in intensity. The esophageal involvement is assumed to precede heart disease in endemic regions. Furthermore, there is a geographical distribution, with the most common digestive form in the South Amazon, predominantly in the Southern Cone countries. [22]

The initial and constant symptom of esophageal involvement in chronic Chagas disease most often is dysphagia. This symptom develops slowly with solid food and requires the intake of liquid (usually water) to facilitate swallowing. The dysphagia then progresses to liquid food and occurs over a variable but generally long period. This symptom is triggered by the cold temperature of the food. Dysphagia may be absent in the early stage of esophageal disease and may decrease in very advanced cases when the megaesophagus becomes a reservoir for food. Frequently, the impaction of pieces of improperly chewed solid food, such as meat, occurs during the transition to the stomach, causing obstruction that may require medical intervention. Other symptoms that accompany dysphagia and have relevance to the clinical diagnosis of chagasic esophagopathy are esophageal pain and regurgitation. The pain may be associated with swallowing food (odynophagia) or may occur spontaneously as a result of spasmodic contractions of the hypersensitive esophagus in response to stimuli. In this case, the contractions simulate cardiac ischemic pain (retrosternal, of great intensity, with sudden onset and possibly constrictive) that radiates to the neck, jaw or back. The pain improves with fluid intake and is not triggered by physical exertion. Regurgitation is delayed, occurs in more severe forms of megaesophagus and is usually related to lying down at bedtime. This condition disrupts sleep and produces cough and aspiration, which may cause pneumonia. Other less specific symptoms are weight loss, heartburn, hiccups, constipation and hypersalivation. Hypersalivation is typical of esophageal diseases due to obstruction; in the case of megaesophagus, this condition is accompanied by hypertrophy of the parotid that generates a characteristic type of face called cat face. Weight loss and malnutrition may occur when food intake is reduced and constipation also may be a consequence associated with megacolon. Chagasic esophagopathy should be differentiated from idiopathic achalasia, which has very similar clinical features. In fact, in endemic regions, positive serology for Chagas disease associated with megacolon and cardiopathy may suggest the diagnosis of chagasic megaesophagus. Radiological testing allows for a confirmation of the diagnosis and classification of the progressive levels of severity. Early effects include a slow transit time and difficulty emptying content of the gastrointestinal tract, which can worsen and lead to megaesophagus [21]. Thus, the esophagogram allows for classification into groups from I, the anectasic forms, to IV, which indicates dolicomegaesophagus. An upper digestive endoscopy is required for all patients with megaesophagus. Although it is not essential for the diagnosis, this exam is intended to exclude other associated pathologic processes that can cause similar symptoms, such as neoplasms. The treatment is palliative and involves a restoration of the transit of food from the esophagus to the stomach because the neuronal denervation is irreversible. These measures include hygienic-dietetic measures generally known and applied by the patients themselves, such as eating slowly, chewing food thoroughly, avoiding solids and facilitating swallowing with water. These patients must avoid cold foods and eating close to bedtime. Medications such as nitrates and calcium channel blockers have been shown to reduce the pressure of the lower esophageal sphincter. Thus, sublingual administration of 5 mg of dinitrate of isosorbitol or 10 mg of nifedipine 15 minutes before main meals was shown to improve dysphagia in a group of patients with chagasic megaesophagus [21]. However, side effects such as headache and hypotension are common, and the patients should be alerted to these effects. Invasive procedures have better long-term results and consist of surgery and dilatation of the lower esophageal sphincter by probes or balloons. The indication depends on the stage of the disease, exceptionally for individuals in group I. In those individuals in groups II and III according to the classification of Rezende [21], both procedures are indicated, sequentially or together, depending on the experience level of the available medical professionals. More aggressive surgical procedures, such as esophagectomy, are indicated for patients in group IV.

Chagas disease affects the distal regions of the colon, especially the rectum, sigmoid colon and descending colon and constipation is the most significant symptom. This symptom develops slowly and gradually and may extend to months of fecal retention. Because of the liquid absorption, feces become hard. This condition accompanies meteorism and rectal dyschezia. Unlike megaesophagus, megacolon may be evidenced in the physical examination at its most severe stage through visualization of the loop in the abdominal wall, usually distended and tympanic, due to the retention of gases. When dilated, the loop may be palpable, revealing an increased diameter and fecal content. The diagnosis is made by contrast radiography of the colon using a barium enema. Standardized tests determine an increase of the diameter of the colon from six cm in the anteroposterior radiographic projection [21]. A digital rectal examination and colonoscopy are part of the subsequent investigation of the chronic constipation, including for cases of chagasic megacolon. Unlike megaesophagus, there is no relationship between megacolon and cancer of the large intestine [20]. Fecaloma, or a fecal tumor, is a complication of megacolon that can be perceived through palpation of the abdomen. This fecal mass is inelastic, with a consistency of clay and the pathognomonic Gersuny sign. The fecalomas that remain in the colon for long periods traumatize the mucus membrane, causing ulcers that may perforate and result in extremely severe fecal peritonitis. In those cases, very large fecal impactions may occur that stop flow by obstructing the intestine, causing acute abdomen. In addition to fecaloma, another complication of the megacolon is intestinal volvulus, which causes acute abdomen due to low intestinal obstruction. The progression of the volvulus is variable, depending on the degree of twisting of the intestinal loop. This condition is benign when incomplete and may be severe when vascular compression and loop necrosis occur. The diagnostic and therapeutic procedures for these situations are those customary for cases of acute abdomen. As for megaesophagus, elective treatment for the megacolon is palliative, consisting of a non-constipating diet, laxative medications and bowel enemas, with variable responses depending on the severity. The fecaloma may require manual removal of the feces under anesthesia. Surgery to resect the dilated region is recommended for cases that do not respond to medical treatment or those with complications. The results are variable, with better responses in the short term, and constipation is often resolved.

In addition to the esophagus and colon, functional changes and expansions in the stomach, duodenum, small intestine, gallbladder and extrahepatic bile ducts have been described. Additionally, there are cases of dilated ureter, urinary bladder and bronchi. In these situations, the clinical features are not as specific as for megaesophagus and megacolon.

Clinical Aspects of Congenital Chagas Disease

Regarding clinical aspects of congenital Chagas disease, up to 90% of patients are asymptomatic, and changes are not detected in clinical examinations [23]. Symptoms may manifest as low birth weight and may result in miscarriage and prematurity. Clinical manifestations may occur within the first days of life or later and overlap with symptoms and signs of the acute phase as described above. However, encephalitis and meningitis are important presentations of congenital Chagas disease that occur early in utero and in the first days or months of life. Development of these conditions is most likely related to the maturing immune system of the fetus and the child, as these manifestations are almost exclusive to these age groups. Due to the possibility of severe clinical conditions associated with high mortality, the diagnosis of congenital Chagas disease should be emphasized, especially in endemic regions for trypanosomiasis. Because of current migratory patterns, the epidemiological history of the mother has an important role even in non-endemic areas [24]. For diagnostic purposes, the direct measurement of *T. cruzi* must be made in the placental cord blood or in blood samples from newborns [10]. The microhematocrit concentration method has been recommended because of its high sensitivity and requirement of only a small amount of blood. If diagnosis by parasitological examination is not possible, a serological diagnosis should be made nine months after birth. In the case of congenital Chagas disease, benznidazole treatment should be instituted as early as possible; this medication has a high efficacy in curing infected patients, with a success rate of 100% when administration is initiated in the first year of life [23]. After treatment, there must be clinical and laboratory follow-up of the patient, with the objective of evaluating the results of treatment. The patients can be considered cured when conventional serology evaluations are persistently negative. All newborns of mothers born or coming from endemic areas for Chagas disease or with a positive epidemiological history should be assessed to allow for early diagnosis and immediate specific treatment for Chagas disease.

Clinical Aspects of Chagas Disease in Immunosuppressed Patients

Immunosuppression originates from various conditions, such as chemotherapy for cancer or for control of organ transplantation rejection, may change the natural evolution of Chagas disease, especially in its chronic phase. Moreover, with the advent of AIDS, the observation of clinical features of Chagas disease in immunosuppressed patients became more frequent [9]. Most people in these situations follow the natural course of trypanosomiasis. Nevertheless, a percentage of the patients (15 to 40%) present clinical aspects of the acute phase of Chagas disease again, especially increased parasitemia by *T. cruzi*, which happens to be detected in direct parasitological examinations in peripheral blood and other body fluids, especially cerebrospinal fluid [8]. This situation has been called reactivation and occurs in individuals with levels of T CD4$^+$ below 200 cells/mm^3, such as with AIDS patients. This condition affects individuals in all stages and clinical forms of Chagas disease, but it has been observed at a higher frequency with serious presentations of meningoencephalitis rather that in the acute stage for immunocompetent patients. The neurological clinical picture reflects intracranial hypertension, motor location, loss of consciousness and seizures, and general systemic manifestations such as fever, poor general condition, etc. Computerized tomography of the brain or nuclear magnetic resonance is essential for the diagnosis of neurological injury, but these exams are nonspecific for Chagas disease. The differential diagnosis should include toxoplasmosis, abscesses, fungal infections, tuberculosis, metastases, lymphoma and progressive multifocal leukoencephalopathy. The definitive diagnosis occurs when *T. cruzi* is found in the cerebrospinal fluid, brain biopsy material or upon necropsy. The other changes observed in the cerebrospinal fluid are nonspecific and compatible with meningitis with light cerebrospinal fluid. The prognosis is severe, with death in 100% of cases that do not receive specific treatment for *T. cruzi*. However, when the diagnosis is quick and treatment is initiated early, the prognosis is greatly improved. Reactivation in the heart can occur, but the diagnosis is more difficult because the clinical features are similar to those of decompensated chronic cardiopathy. Additionally, the reactivation has been described elsewhere, such as in the skin, peritoneum, pericardium, duodenum and uterus, but without the complications observed in the central nervous system [9].

Final Considerations

The clinical features of Chagas disease are wide-ranging and variable, depending on the stage and the clinical forms presented by individuals at the time of medical attention. The acute stage reflects systemic manifestations of a general response to the parasite. The chronic stage is characterized by mechanisms that depend on the parasite and on the host-parasite interaction, especially the specific immunologic response. The indeterminate form does not show any clinical manifestations due to an adapted host-parasite interaction and the majority of individuals in endemic regions have this form.

The predominant clinical features of cardiopathy are of minor severity, including intraventricular blocks and lower expression arrhythmias. Electrocardiogram examination remains the best and most cost-effective test. However, ventricular dysfunction and severe arrhythmias occur more frequently than in other cardiopathies and are predictive of a poor prognosis and death. Megaesophagus and megacolon occur less frequently, and mortality is lower, but morbidity is high; furthermore, there is no definitive therapy for these conditions. Great progress has been achieved in the identification of clinical features, diagnostic ability, and therapeutic strategies since the first description of the disease, but challenges remain, especially related to validation of risk stratification, to new technologies to be applied and to controlled prospective studies specific for individuals with Chagas disease.

References

[1]   Pinto Dias JC. Globalização, iniqüidade e doença de Chagas. *Cad Saúde Pública. 2007*; 23(Supl): 513-22.

[2]   Akhavan D. Analise de custo-efetividade do programa de controle da doença de Chagas no Brasil. Relatório final. *Organização Pan-Americana da Saúde*. 2000; Brasília/Brasil, 271 pp.

[3]   Castro JÁ, de Mecca MM, Bartel LC. Toxic effects of drugs used to treat Chagas'disease (American trypanosomiasis). *Hum Exp Toxicol*. 2006; 25(8):471-79

[4]   Urbina JA. Chemotherapy of Chagas'disease: the how and the why. *J Mol Med*. 1999; 77: 332-38.

[5]   Relatório técnico do Ministério da Saúde, Brasil, 2006: OMS/OPAS-*Certificação do Brasil como área interrompida de transmissão da doença de chagas pelo Triatoma. infestans*.

[6]   Chagas C. *Tripanosomíase americana: forma aguda da moléstia*. Mem Inst Oswaldo Cruz. 1916; 8: 37-65.

[7]   Lugones H, Ledesma O, Storino R, Marteleur A, Meneclier C, Barbieri G. Chagas Agudo. In: Storino R, Milei J editors. Enfermedad *de Chagas. Doyma Argentina S.A.* 1994; 209-34.

[8]   Almeida EA, Lima JN, Lages-Silva E, Guariento ME, Aoki FH, Torres-Morales AE. Chagas'disease and HIV co-infection in patients without effective antiretroviral therapy: prevalence, clinical presentation and natural history. *Trans Royal Soc Trop Med and Hyg*. 2010; 104: 447-52.

[9] Almeida EA, Ramos Jr NA, Correia D, Shikanai-Yassuda MA. Co-infection *Trypanosoma cruzi*/HIV: systematic review (1980-2010). *Braz Soc Trop Med.* 2011; 44(6): 755-63.

[10] Consenso Brasileiro em Doença de Chagas. *J Braz Soc Trop Med.* 2005; 38(Supl III):14-5.

[11] Prata A. Clinical and epidemiological aspects of Chagas disease. *The Lancet Infect Dis.* 2001; 1: 92-100.

[12] Rassi Jr A, Rassi A, Rassi SG. Predictors of mortality in chronic Chagas'disease. A systematic review of observational studies. *Circulation.* 2007; 6: 1101-08.

[13] Terzi FVO, Siqueira Filho AG, Nascimento EM, Pereira BB, Pedrosa RC. Regional left ventricular dysfunction and its association with complex ventricular arrhythmia, in chagasic patients with normal or borderline electrocardiogram. *J Braz Soc Trop Med.* 2010; 43(5): 557-61.

[14] Pedrosa RC, Campos MC. Exercise testing and 24 hours Holter monitoring in the detection of complex ventricular arrhytmias in different stages of chronic Chagas' heart disease. *J Braz Soc Trop Med.* 2004; 37(5): 376-83.

[15] I Diretriz Latino-Americana para o Diagnóstico e Tratamento da Cardiopatia Chagásica. *Arq Bras Cardiol.* 2011; 97(Supl 3):18-22.

[16] Rassi A, Rassi Jr A, Rassi SG, Rassi AG. Cardiopatia crônica: arritmias. In Dias, JCP, Coura JR editors. Clínica e terapêutica da doença de Chagas. *Editora Fiocruz, Brasil*; 1997; 201-15.

[17] Rassi Jr A, Rassi A, Marin-Neto JA. Chagas' heart disease: pathophysiologic mechanism, prognostic factors and risk stratification. *Mem Inst Oswaldo Cruz.* 2009; 104: 152-58.

[18] Baroldi G, Oliveira SJM, Silver MD. Sudden and unexpected death in clinically 'silent' Chagas' disease. A hypothesis. *Internat J Cardiol.* 1997; 58: 263-68.

[19] Pimenta J, Valente N, Miranda M. Long-term follow-up of asymptomatic chagasic individuals with intraventricular conduction disturbances, correlating with non-chagasic patients. *J Braz Soc Trop Med.* 1999; 32(6): 621-31.

[20] Rassi Jr A, Rassi A, Marin-Neto JA. Chagas disease. *The Lancet.* 2010; 375(17):1388-1401.

[21] Rezende JM. O aparelho digestivo na doença de Chagas-Aspectos clínicos. In Dias, JCP, Coura, JR editors. Clínica e terapêutica da doença de Chagas. *Editora Fiocruz, Brasil*; 1997; 153-76.

[22] Coura JR, Borges-Pereira J. Chagas' disease. What is known and what should be improved: a systemic review. *J Braz Soc Trop Med.* 2012; 45(3): 286-96.

[23] Carlier Y, Torrico F. Congenital infection with *Trypanosoma cruzi*: from mechanisms of transmission to estrategies for diagnosis and control. *J Braz Soc Trop Med.* 2003; 36(6): 767-71.

[24] Basile L, Oliveira I, Plasencia A. A working group for developing the Catalonian Screening Programe for congenital transmission of Chagas disease. The current escreening programme for congenital transmission of Chagas disease in Catalonia, Spain. Euro Surveill, 16(38): 19972, 2011. Available online: *http://www.eurosurveillance.org/ViewArticle.*

In: Chagas Disease   ISBN: 978-1-62808-681-2
Editors: F. R. Gadelha, E.d.F. Peloso   © 2013 Nova Science Publishers, Inc.

Chapter V

Clinical and Laboratory Diagnosis

Marta de Lana
Full Professor - Faculty of Pharmacy
Universidade Federal de Ouro Preto, Ouro-Preto-MG, Brazil

Abstract

For the successful clinical and laboratory diagnosis of Chagas disease, the first consideration is the patient's phase of infection. The clinical signals, symptoms and physiological alterations, as well as the laboratory data/features, are well correlated with the natural clinical evolution of the disease. While in the beginning stages of the infection (acute phase) some patients present several severe clinical alterations, the great majority of patients are asymptomatic (95%) or oligosymptomatic, thus making clinical diagnosis difficult. On the other hand, laboratory examinations, such as specific IgM or IgG-antibody assays for *Trypanosoma cruzi* conducted with conventional serological tests (IIF, ELISA and IHR) and parasitological tests (especially fresh blood examination, blood smear and concentration methods), allow definitive diagnosis. Following the acute phase, the disease evolves to the subacute phase. During this phase, all symptoms and clinical signs progressively disappear, with rare exceptions. When patients progress to the chronic phase, after approximately six to nine months of infection, the disease evolves to an indeterminate or asymptomatic clinical form. At this phase of infection, the only diagnosis possibility is laboratory-based conventional serological tests that employ specific antigens of *T. cruzi* for the detection of IgG antibodies, which are always present in infected patients. Parasitological tests (xenodiagnosis, hemoculture, polymerase chain reaction (PCR) may be used at this phase, but they display low sensitivity because of low and subpatent parasitemia due to the specific immune response of the host against the parasite. In the chronic and symptomatic patients, conventional serology and cardiac and gastrointestinal electrophysiological tests are fundamental for definitive diagnosis, evaluation of the clinical evolution and prognosis of the disease. One important feature of Chagas disease diagnosis is that when patients present the indeterminate form of the disease, serological tests are the only proof of infection; thus, these tests need to be properly conducted. In this chapter, the fundamental specific clinical and laboratory diagnostic methods are described for each phase and clinical form of Chagas disease, following its natural clinical evolution. In addition, the diagnosis procedures applied to particular situations, including cure control, blood donor screening, congenital transmission, immunosuppressed patients and others, are described.

Introduction

The great majority of the methodologies for the diagnosis of Chagas disease is used only in specialized laboratories for research and consequently cannot be applied by public health services and/or clinical analysis laboratories due to their complexity and time-consuming nature. This is a consequence of the complexity of Chagas disease infection. The infection phase when the parasite is easily detected (acute phase) is short, but the clinical suspicion is often not possible because the majority of the patients are oligosymptomatic. However, during the chronic phase of the infection, which may last the patient's lifetime, the detection of the etiological agent is limited and difficult because parasitemia is low and the best methods for diagnosis are performed only in research laboratories. PCR (polymerase chain reaction), although important for demonstrating the presence of parasite DNA and, consequently, helping with the etiological diagnosis, cannot be used in isolation. Thus, the diagnostic tools generally applied in clinical laboratories are based on serological tests. Several of these tests are available, and the careful choice of reagents and methods are fundamental in aiding physicians to make an accurate diagnosis, after taking into account anamnesis and the clinical patient signals. In addition, several other particularities have to be considered for the correct diagnosis, such as the mechanism of infection, immune status of the patient, simultaneous infection, cure control and blood donor screening.

Acute Phase Diagnosis

Clinical Diagnosis

T. cruzi infection can be acquired, as described in chapter XX, via several mechanisms. These different possibilities, associated with the first cells/ organ infected and inoculum, result in different clinical pictures during the acute phase. The presence of the entry signals, as Romaña signal [1] and/or chagoma of inoculation [2] respectively, greatly aid in establishing clinical suspicion of Chagas disease. In addition, the patient origin, which is associated to satellite or generalized adenopathy, hepatosplenomegaly, tachycardia, generalized edema or edema of the feet, can lead to suspicion that the patient is in the acute phase of Chagas disease. Myocarditis is a central pathological disorder that, when intense, can cause cardiac failure and contribute to a poor prognosis. Neurological perturbations are rare and the consequence of the meningoencephalitis that occurs in young children and immunosuppressed patients is severe.

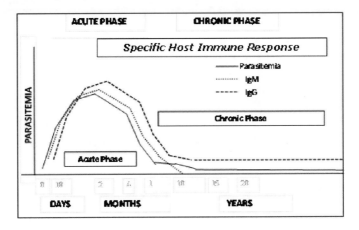

Figure 1. Evolution of *Trypanosoma cruzi* infection in mammals. Acute phase (high parasitemia) and Chronic phase (low parasitemia).

In general, clinical diagnosis of the disease in its acute phase is not successful because a high percentage of the patients are asymptomatic or oligosymptomatic. It is difficult to diagnose these patients because they display several symptoms very similar to other infectious fever diseases. Except for electrocardiogram (ECG), the battery of examinations normally used for the diagnosis of the chronic phase (chest X-ray and barium contrast of the gastrointestinal tract (GIT) may present normal results during the acute phase.

Laboratory Diagnosis

Various laboratory diagnosis methods can be applied to this phase of the infection. These methods can be classified as parasitological (mandatory at this phase) and serological. In the acute phase occur higher parasitemia, the presence of unspecific antibodies and the initial appearance of specific antibodies (IgM and IgG) that increase in level progressively throughout the acute phase of the infection (Figure 1).

Direct Parasitological Methods

The direct parasitological methods are more often used in the acute phase of the infection because the parasitemia is higher and more easily detectable than during the chronic phase (when the specific immune response of the host against the infection is present) (Figure 1).

Fresh blood examination: This method consists of the examination of a volume of 5 µl of peripheral blood collected from a fingertip, foot, ear or vein. The blood is covered with a coverslip and examined via microscopy [3]. This method is used for the daily quantification of the parasitemia. Refringent blood trypomastigotes are observed moving quickly between the blood cells and platelets. The detection of only one moving parasite provides a definitive diagnosis without need for other examinations.

Thick smear: This method, typically used for the diagnosis of malaria, can also be used in the acute phase of Chagas disease, but its sensitivity is lower than a fresh blood examination. For this examination, a drop of blood is distributed in a circle via circular movements of the glass slide, dried, fixed with ethanol and stained. The visualization and identification of the parasite is more difficult than with other parasitological methods due to blood concentration, disruption of red blood cells and the release of hemoglobin.

Dry smear: This method offers an advantage because the observation of the parasite morphology is easier than the other methods described. On the other hand, its use offers good results only when the parasitemia is very higher (> 500,000 trypomastigotes/0.1 ml of blood). In both the *thick smear* and *dry smear* techniques, the preparations have to be fixed with methanol before being stained with Romanowsky dyes.

Concentration Methods

Microhematocrit: For this method, only 100 µl of blood is collected directly in a heparinized capillary tube. The tube is immediately centrifuged in a hematocrit centrifuge. Parasites may be seen in the intermediary layer between the red blood cells and plasma, directly on the inverted microscope. Although it has a risk of accidental contamination, the capillary can be broken at this layer and a drop of the leukocyte cream examined via microscope. In addition, this method is highly sensitive and particularly applicable to congenital infections.

Leukocyte Cream: For this method, a volume of 3-5 mL of heparinized blood is collected in a centrifuged tube and centrifuged. The parasites may be sought, via microscopy, in a drop of the leukocyte layer on a glass slide covered with a cover slip.

Strout Method: This method is similar to the leukocyte cream examination but is more complex and the blood is collected without anticoagulant. Thus, the blood has to be clotted at room temperature or more quickly at 37° C. The parasites escape the clot of the blood exudates, which is double centrifuged. A drop of this sediment is examined in microscope on a glass slide covered with a cover slip.

Indirect Parasitological Methods

Blood inoculation in mice: The inoculation of a volume of 0.3 mL of blood or 0.3-0.5 mL of leukocyte cream or serum is used for the intraperitoneal inoculation of young or immunosuppressed mice, especially from isogenic lineages sensitive to *T. cruzi* infection that may reveal the infection later. Thus, mice should be examined daily one week post-inoculation. The parasites, if present, can be found in fresh blood examination.

Xenodiagnosis and Hemoculture: These methods will be further described in this chapter. Although these methods are very sensitive in the acute phase of the infection (100%), they are not normally indicated for acute cases because approximately 30 days are necessary for a positive test result, and these patients need to be immediately etiologically treated (compulsory treatment).

Blood culture or biopsy culture material: Blood or biopsy materials from lymphnodes can be cultured to facilitate parasite growth [4].

Serological Tests

Serological diagnostic tests are applicable in both the acute and chronic phases of the infection because the tests used in this context detect specific antibodies (IgG and IgM) in the serum of the patient. Serological tests can be performed with serum, plasma and in blood collected directly in filter paper. Serum and plasma must be stored at -20 °C after separated by centrifugation of the whole blood. Samples collected in filter paper must be dried at room temperature and stored in a refrigerator. In this case, the test must be performed within one to two months to avoid antibody titer decrease. Alternatively, urine [5] and pericardial fluid [6] can be used for the diagnosis with the methodologies of the serological tests, as well as punctures of organs or tissues where the amastigote stage of the parasite, inflammatory lesions or eventually fibrosis might be observed. These possibilities are applicable for certain clinical conditions and in experimental animal models.

It is important to keep in mind that, unlike the parasitological methods, the serological tests indicate only the probability of patient infection. Thus, the origin and clinical characteristics of the patient have to be considered for the final diagnosis and, when possible, the parasitological methods are indicated to confirm etiology. Parasitological methods are mandatory during the acute phase because their positivity is high and the etiological treatment of patients with recent infection offers a great probability of parasitological cure, unlike during later chronic infection [7].

During the acute phase, both classes of antibodies, IgM and IgG, are present in concentrations that vary throughout the time of infection (Figure 1). IgM appears earlier than IgG, and both can be detected after two weeks of infection at increasing levels during the acute phase. The techniques frequently used to detect the antibodies include IIF (Indirect Immunofluorescence) or ELISA (Enzyme-linked-immunosorbent-assay).

With the progression of the infection, the IgM antibodies decrease until their disappearance (with some exceptions), and the IgG-based specific immune response is active and easily detectable after two months of infection. The IgG levels also increase progressively. IgG remains elevated for a longer period than IgM in the acute phase and decreases progressively until it stabilizes; however, unlike IgM, the IgG antibodies never disappear and therefore Chagas-related antibodies can be detected for the lifetime of the patient.

Chronic Phase Diagnosis

In the chronic phase of Chagas disease lower parasitemia and the presence of specific antibodies (mainly IgG) are observed at higher concentrations in the majority of patients examined by IIF reaction [8]. During this phase, IgM antibodies are sporadically detected at low titers. The conventional serological tests or indirect parasitological tests are recommended for the diagnosis of the chronic phase of Chagas disease. The more commonly used serological tests are ELISA, Indirect hemagglutination reaction (IHR) and IIF tests. Xenodiagnosis, hemoculture and inoculation of patient's blood into laboratory animals are the most commonly used parasitological methods during this phase. These methods are specifically necessary when the serology is discordant or in monitoring of treatment efficacy.

Clinical Diagnosis

The clinical diagnosis of the chronic phase of Chagas disease is dependent on the clinical form presented by the patient. In general, in the majority of infected patients (50 to 70%), a clinical diagnosis is not possible because the patients present the indeterminate form of the disease. The only indication of the infection is via conventional serology (always positive) or by the demonstration of the parasite by the less sensitive parasitological tests (hemoculture, xenodiagnosis), PCR and others. For the clinical and physical examinations, conventional ECG and thorax X-ray plus esophagus and colon barium-contrasted X-ray are employed [9]. These evaluations permit the classification of the patients as indeterminate, cardiac, digestive or mixed form of the disease [10]. Only more accurate examinations, such as ergometric test, Holter monitoring, echocardiogram and myocardium scintigraphy, may detect the alterations that are imperceptible during common clinical evaluations.

From the didactic point of view, patients with the cardiac form of the disease may present different levels of physiological alterations. They can be classified as cardiac mild, moderate and severe. Patients may be asymptomatic or present congestive syndrome and/or alterations of cardiac rhythm and/or electric stimuli conduction. Mild cardiopathy includes patients without complaints of cardiac failure and/or arrhythmias and normal cardiac area. Observed ECG alterations are primarily disturbances of conduction, ventricular repolarization and extrasystoles. In some cases, there is a surprising scarcity of symptoms associated with the electrocardiographic signals and anatomopathological lesions. Moderate cardiopathy includes patients with arrhythmias or cardiac insufficiency. The principal symptomatology includes palpitation and dyspnea of effort. In addition, the patients may experience arrhythmias and extrasystoles followed by systolic blow and hypophonic cardiac sounds. The cardiac X-ray area may be increased and sudden death may occur. Patients with severe cardiopathy predominantly present symptoms of congestive cardiac failure. The peripheral edema, ascites, hepatosplenomegaly and increased jugular venous pressure are more remarkable than the pulmonary congestion. Systemic or pulmonary embolisms originating from endocardial mural thrombi are frequent and sometimes severe, even in the absence of cardiac insufficiency. When cardiac decompensation manifests, the patient may or not recuperate and survive with sustained cardiac insufficiency until new decompensation episodes. After one year of initial decompensation, death occurs in approximately 50% of cases. Sudden or expected death may occur.

Laboratory Diagnosis

Parasitological Tests

Indirect parasitological tests are applicable during the chronic phase of Chagas disease because parasitemia is subpatent and scarce. The principle of the techniques used is to give the opportunity for a parasite obtained from the patient to multiply in triatomines (xenodiagnosis), artificial culture medium (hemoculture) or animal models (inoculation in mice). As these techniques are not evaluating the parasites directly in the patient, they are called indirect parasitological methods. They are the only methods that, in fact and undoubtedly do the etiologic diagnosis of Chagas disease.

Xenodiagnosis: It can be natural, using uninfected triatomines for direct feeding of patient blood, or artificial, when the patient's blood is previously collected with an anticoagulant and then offered to the triatomines using a special device [11-15]. This method is specifically indicated when the patient is allergic to triatomine bites and its saliva; or in experimental studies with standardized inocula. In recent years, the artificial method has become more frequently used than the natural one, and it sometimes offers better results because the insects feed better [13]. Based on the principle of parasite-host interaction, it is recommended that the triatomine species used should have the same geographic origin of the patient. The steps of the xenodiagnosis are as follows [12]: forty nymphs of the third, fourth or fifth instars of triatomines, depending on the size of the triatomine species, and free of *T. cruzi* infection, are separated into four boxes with ten specimens each. Each box is covered with a membrane, and the insects are put in contact with the arms, legs or back of the patient for blood sucking for approximately 30 min. After feeding, they are stored and examined 30, 60 or 90 days later. The examination may be individual or grouped (10 or 40 insects). The insects are subjected to abdominal compression, and the intestinal content is collected and examined with a microscope. It is highly advisable to consider the potential presence of *Blastocrithidae triatominae* and *Trypanosoma rangeli* [16].

The sensitivity of this method ranges from 30 to 70% and may be increased by performing total dissection of the intestines of the insects, followed by examination of the whole intestinal content. The results are expressed as the number of insects with flagellates or, in experimental studies, as the number of epimastigotes or trypomastigotes by insect.

The principal limitations of this technique are its time-consuming nature and the need for triatomines free of *T. cruzi* infection, possible only in a specialized laboratory. This method is laborious and also offers a risk of accidental transmission of the infection, especially during the examination of the insects. Xenodiagnosis positivity is lowest in patients undergoing monitoring for etiological treatment efficacy.

Hemoculture: Briefly, [17] 30 mL of venous blood is collected with heparin from adults, centrifuged, and the plasma layer is separated for culture in liquid medium (LIT) [18]. The blood cells are washed in LIT medium and the superior layer of leucocytes is carefully removed and transferred to a tube for culture in LIT. The microscopic examinations may be performed every 15 or 30 days for at least 90 days, using a drop of the intermediary layer of the culture in contact with the sediment of cells or cells degradation. The results may be expressed as the number of positive tubes and the time elapsed after culture. This technique can reach 55 to 79% of positivity. However, when hemoculture and xenodiagnosis are used in parallel the positivity increases.

PCR: This method is based on the detection of kDNA (most common), nuclear DNA or RNA of *T. cruzi* previously extracted from the patient sample. PCR may be applied to blood samples, tissue (biopsies) and fluid as well as to intestinal contents of triatomines. It has been verified that as a consequence of the scarce and intermittent nature of the parasitemia, especially in chronic or etiologically treated patients, this technique presents variable sensitivity dependent on the type of the parasite present or predominant in the patient. On many occasions, this technique is the only method to provide a positive result in *T. cruzi* serological-positive patients, as it is able to detect one fentogram of DNA present in a sample [19]. A positive PCR result is indicative of infection, but a negative PCR must be believed only if other serological and parasitological tests are also negative [20].

Serological Tests

The principle of conventional serological tests is based on the detection of specific antibodies that recognize *T. cruzi* antigens. The antibodies are immunoglobulins raised against the parasite's surface antigens or internal antigens released in the blood stream of the host throughout the infection or after disintegration of the parasites. These antigens are originated from different parasite stages allowing the diagnosis of the infection during all stages of infection. *Shed acute phase antigen* (SAPA) is an antigen released by the parasites, and it is present mainly during the acute phase of the infection [21]. *Trypomastigotes excreted-secreted antigens* (TESA-cruzi antigens), an antigen derived from trypomastigotes in cell culture, offers good results in discordant serology situations [22].

Antigen Variety for Serological Tests

Regardless of the *T. cruzi* strain used, there is a tendency that some country or geographical region uses an antigen representative of the local predominant parasite lineage. However, the literature indicates numerous particularities linked to the distinct *T. cruzi* lineages, including antigenicity and the ability to induce the formation of antibodies detectable by serological tests [23, 24]. Thus, it has been demonstrated that two (TcI and TcII) of the six genetic groups or discrete typing units (DTUs) more widely spread are antigenically distinct and represent the majority of the *T. cruzi* isolates [25]. The standardized and available serological tests (IIF, ELISA and IHR) use the antigenic preparation of Y strain cultivated in LIT medium.

One important problem regarding the use of serological tests for Chagas disease diagnosis is cross-reaction with other etiological agents. This happens especially with other species of the Trypanosomatidae family [26]. As American Trypanosomiasis occurs in Central and South America simultaneously with parasites from the genus *Leishmania*, this constitutes an important limitation of the common serological tests. Exploring methodological particularities of the ELISA test with serial serum dilutions [27] it was verified that with total IgG at a dilution 1:320, is possible to distinguish Chagas disease from Visceral Leishmaniasis, American Tegumentary Leishmaniasis, Syphilis, Hepatitis C Virus and HIV. Similarly, cross-reaction is common with *T. rangeli* spread throughout Latin America [26]. However, the use of PCR with specific primers distinguishes these species [28].

Conventional Serological Tests

The commonly used test for the serodiagnosis of Chagas disease is the Complement Fixation Reaction (CFR) [29] followed by the IIF [30]. CRF is rarely used. The main problems of all these methodologies are related to the different sources and preparations of antigens as well as the differences in methodology by distinct manufacturer. This reality led to the publication of manuals for good laboratory practices by the Brazilian Health Ministry [31].

The principal characteristics of the serological tests are specificity and sensitivity. The specificity is the capability of the test to detect all cases without the infection (absence of false positive) while the sensitivity is the capability of the test to detect all infected cases (absence of false negative). There is no test 100% specific and sensitive. To improve the specificity and sensibility, several measures are used: the simultaneous use of more than one test with different antigens and/or reaction mechanisms, the use of good positive and negative control samples, repetition of the tests with the same sample or with other samples from the same patient, continuous training of the technicians, quality control program regularly applied by internal or external personnel or public services.

Indirect Immunofluorescence (IIF): This technique allows the use of specific conjugates and has high sensitivity when performed by a skilled technician (98%). IIF is indicated for the diagnosis of acute phase and congenital transmission of Chagas disease. Briefly, specific anti-*T. cruzi* antibodies react with the epimastigote form of the parasite previously fixed on a microscope slide. Next, the sample is incubated in specific conditions so that the corresponding conjugate labeled with a fluorescent reagent is able to recognize the complex antigen-antibody already present. Immunofluorescent microscopy is necessary to verify the fluorescence of positive samples.

A reactivity ≥ 1:40 dilution is considered positive. The disadvantages of this method are that the quality of the antigens as well as of the other reagents, including the pH of the glycerol used in the preparation of the reaction for microscope reading. Most patients present reactivity higher than 1:40.

Enzyme-linked-immunosorbent-assay (ELISA): As IIF, this method also detects different classes of immunoglobulin and has the same indications. Its reaction mechanism is based on the detection of an antigen-antibody complex by a conjugate with specific anti-*T. cruzi* antibodies. The results are interpreted by reading colored enzymatic reactions in a spectrophotometer. Epidemiological inquiry is a particular application of this technique because it allows the testing of a great number of samples simultaneously and can be used with sera samples fixed in filter paper [32]. However, the reactive cases or gray zone cases (± 10% around the cut off) must also be confirmed using conventional serological tests (at least two tests with concordant results). Due to the ease of ELISA implementation, its ability to be automated and the fact that conjugates for different classes and subclasses of immunoglobulins can be used, several antigenic preparations, synthetic and non-synthetic, have been evaluated with this method. One of the most important contributions has been offered by the use of recombinant antigens and the results are variable depending of their composition, source or combinations. One important combination of recombinant antigens (H49, JL7, A13, B13, JL8, and 1F8) is the ability to distinguish Chagas disease from leishmaniasis [33].

Indirect Hemagglutination Reaction (IHR): This technique is the most simple and fast (one or two hours) among the serological tests and the most used in clinical laboratories due to easy handling and the lack of need for specialized equipment. Briefly, sera samples are mixed with animal red blood cells (rabbits, chicken or other species) previously sensitized with *T. cruzi* antigens of distinct preparations originating from several countries, particularly Brazil, Argentina and Chile. In the presence of anti-*T. cruzi* antibodies the red blood cells agglutinate and the visual reading of the reaction is very simple. Several types of kits are commercially available, and therefore, the sensitivity and specificity of the reaction are variable. There are also difficulties establishing a cut off with the visual reading of the reaction. In general, the specificity is high, but the sensitivity (< 20% relatively) depends on the manufacturer. Thus, this method should be used in parallel with other previously described methods for better confirmation of the diagnosis as recommended [65]. Although IHR offers several advantages, the nonspecific reactions are possible (natural antibodies that react with the red blood cells of the species of animal used).

The use of at least two serological tests with distinct principles to confirm a diagnosis of Chagas disease is recommended [34]. If the results are discordant, the repetition of both tests is recommended; if the discordance remains, a third test with different principles is indicated.

In some cases, it may be necessary to perform a fourth test or to perform the reaction in another reference laboratory or employ a non-serological method (parasitological tests), associated if necessary.

Serological Methods not Routinely Used

Western blotting: One example of this methodology is the TESA-blot ELISA, which uses the secreted trypomastigotes antigen [22] more recently introduced for *T. cruzi* diagnosis.

rCRP ELISA: A new approach for diagnosis being explored is the use of a 160-kDa recombinant protein (rCRP) that reacts with complement protein during the phenomenon of complement-mediated lysis (CML) [35, 36].

Rapid test: The Chagas Stat-Pack (CSP) test is one example of a rapid and simple test, practical for routine primary diagnostic use in endemic rural areas or poor communities suffering Chagas disease.

In Bolivia, this test has offered high sensitivity and specificity in the diagnosis of the infection in pregnant women and newborns of mothers infected with *T. cruzi* [37]. This kind of test is very important in blood transfusion in emergency situations.

Common Problems with Serological Testing

There are several common problems with serological tests, including the presence of excess unspecific antibodies that prevent the specific reaction in low dilutions of the serum, such as an excess of IgM that prevents the IgG reaction and rheumatoid factor (especially in immunosuppressed or older patients) when IgM is being evaluated.

In addition, cross-reaction with other parasites such as *Leishmania* sp. or other Trypanosomatidae, toxoplasmosis, schistosomiasis, malaria and others are also an issue.

Non-Conventional Serological Tests

Several laboratory methods are available for monitoring the post-therapeutic Chagas disease cure of patients, including two major categories: parasitological (microhematocrit, xenodiagnostic, hemoculture and PCR) and serological (conventional: ELISA, IIF, IHR and non-conventional: CML, and flow cytometric analysis of anti-live trypomastigote antibodies, FC-ALTA). The long time required for seroreversion after etiologic treatment of *T.cruzi* infection is very slow (10 to 30 years) and seems to be strongly associated with the type and length of infection. This lengthy seroreversion time represents a major drawback of these methods (Table 1).

Table 1. Correlation between the type and length of the infection with the therapeutic effectiveness and the time required for seroreversion after etiological treatment of Chagas disease [source 38, 39]

Type of infection	Length of infection (years)	% of cure	Time required for seroreversion (years)
Congenital transmission	0 – 1	100	100
Recent Acute Phase	1 – 5	60	60
Recent Chronic Phase	12 – 14	60	60
Late Chronic Phase	> 15	0 – 20	0 – 20

This lengthy seroreversion time might be explained by the existence of several mechanisms of auto-immunity in Chagas disease and the longer persistence time of the memory antibodies, among others. It has also been verified that oscillating results from conventional serological tests may indicate that the patient has been cured, which is usually associated with negative PCR and/or non-conventional method results.

A new method to detect anti-live trypomastigote IgG based on flow cytometry technology [40] consists of an indirect immunofluorescence approach using the flow cytometer to increase sensitivity. The result is expressed in percentage of positive fluorescent parasites (PPFP). Despite no direct correlation being observed between the PPFP values and the % of lysis in CML, a strong categorical association was reached between FC-ALTA and CML. The results confirmed the existence of three categories of treated patients similar to those obtained using CML. Following it was standardized a new flow cytometry-based methodology to assess post-therapeutic Chagas disease cure of patients [41]. This method used pre-fixed *T. cruzi* epimastigotes in a multiwell plate (FC-AFEA). All these methods (CML, FC-ALTA and FC-AFEA) have been proposed as a putative methodology for early determination of therapeutic efficacy, especially in animal models, since in human the conventional serology may remain positive for several years post-cure [35]. Table 2 summarizes a provisional proposal to classify Chagas disease patients according to their profiles on parasitological and serological tests applied after etiological treatment. Four major categories can be identified: treated not cured (TNC); treated cured (TC); dissociated (DIS) and inconclusive (INC).

Table 2. Post-therapeutic classification of treated Chagas disease patients according to the results of the parasitological and serological laboratory tests. Source: *[35] and [39]; **[42]

Results Interpretation	Parasitological Tests	Conventional (ELISA, IFI, HAI)	Non-Conventional (C^OML, FC-ALTA)
Treated Not Cured (TNC)*	Pos/Neg	Pos	Pos
Cured (CUR)*	Neg	Neg	Neg
Dissociated (DIS)**	Neg	Pos	Neg
Inconclusive (INC)	Neg	Pos/Neg	Pos/Neg

The general consensus is that serological methods can be used as a criterion to detect therapeutic failure at any phase of the disease and, therefore, are able to identify treated, not cured patients when both conventional and non-conventional serological tests are positive, despite the results of parasitological tests [35, 39]. There is also an overall agreement to identify treated and cured patients as those with negative parasitological and negative serological tests [39, 43]. However, divergent opinions still exist regarding the evaluation of therapeutic effectiveness, since treated patients can display positive/oscillating conventional serology, despite persistent negative results on parasitological and non-conventional serology tests. It has been proposed that these patients, referred as dissociated [35], may also be considered cured, since they present evidence of post-therapeutic cure due their persistently negative parasitological and non-conventional serological tests despite their residual positive conventional serology as a consequence of the long period required for seroreversion, especially when treatment is applied during chronic disease [20, 35, 43].

New approaches have been already carried out using novel antigenic preparations adapted to conventional serology tests. The use of antigens analogue or correspondent to the 160 kDa protein recognized by the lytic antibodies have been already tested [44]. If authors studying patients from other geographical regions corroborate these results, the industrialization of ELISA kits employing recombinant antigens correspondent to the 160 kDa protein offers good potential as a method of evaluating post-treatment cure and could lead to the abolition of the use of more complex methodologies. Moreover, the use of other antigenic targets, including the combined recombinant antigens CRA+FRA [45], have shown promise in the context of cure criterion for Chagas disease.

Taking into account the aforementioned considerations, it is important to ask several important questions in the context of cure criterion in Chagas disease. Is it necessary to wait for the seroreversion of conventional serology to verify the post-therapeutic curing of Chagas disease? Will the residual positive conventional serology persist even after the elimination of the parasites? Can the negative parasitological and non-conventional serological methods attest post-therapeutic cure in Chagas disease? The answers to these questions continue to stimulate the search for novel methodological approaches.

Diagnostic Particularities to Be Considered

Screening of blood donors: Blood transfusion is considered the second most important risk factor for Chagas disease infection. This risk was considerable in Brazil in the 1970s and 1980s and the beginning of the 1990s. Due to this risk, the screening of blood donors for *T. cruzi*, HIV, HVB, HVC and syphilis is performed in Latin America countries, especially in Brazil, Argentina, Honduras, Uruguay and Venezuela [46]. The probability of an individual acquiring *T. cruzi* infection via contaminated blood was estimated to be 20% [47]. Naturally, this risk increases with the number of transfusions received, as is the case of hemophiliacs or individuals with other hematological problems. It is very important to consider that blood transfusion has played a considerable role in the dissemination of Chagas disease in other countries due to the migration of infected patients originating from areas where the screening of blood donors for *T. cruzi* is not performed [48]. The USA, France and Spain are more advanced in the control of Chagas disease as a consequence of better health service and great amounts of immigration from Latin American countries [49, 50]. In practice, the process of screening consists of the elimination of all donors that have at least one conventional serology positive test for *T. cruzi*. The recommendation is the use of at least two serological tests relying on different principles where the ELISA, IIF and IHR are the most frequently used. For security, the simultaneous use of different tests and the evaluation of one serum dilution below the dilution used for the diagnosis are recommended. In some countries, the blood screening service covers all regions; in other cover only the endemic areas. Unfortunately, some evaluations of blind sera panels by different blood services of the same or distinct countries revealed variable percentage of false-negative results [51, 52].

Congenital transmission: The congenital transmission of Chagas disease has played an important role in the transmission of Chagas disease, especially after the implementation of vector control programs in South and Central America and the aforementioned blood screening of donors. Congenital transmission has also been demonstrated around the world [53]. It is important to keep in mind that the same woman may transmit the infection to fetuses in more than one pregnancy throughout her life. Interestingly, only one newborn twin from an infected woman may be infected. A diagnosis of congenital transmission must be performed as soon as possible after birth. However, several characteristics of the mother, such as infection phase, immune status, genetic group of the parasite, the level of parasitemia [54, 55] and several attributes of the newborn such as the period of the pregnancy when the infection was acquired and, consequently, the maturity of his immune system, have important influences on the difficulty of the diagnosis. When the diagnosis of the infection is concluded, notification is mandatory as recommended by WHO and the Brazilian Health Ministry, and the etiological treatment must begin immediately, as the possibility of parasitological cure is high (70 to 100%) at this particular period of the infection. In addition, the disease can be fatal in newborn or lead to other health problems [56].

The rates of congenital transmission vary from country to country and region to region [57, 58] and are apparently related to the degree of area endemicity. Some studies using molecular parasite characterization have demonstrated that all the genetic groups, except TcIII, are associated with congenital transmission [59, 60]. The parasitemia level of the mother may also be related to the parasite genetic group, along with the infection period and immunological status of both the mother and child. Congenital patients may be asymptomatic, oligosymptomatic or fully symptomatic. This makes clinical evaluation of congenital Chagas disease difficult. The main clinical characteristics of infected newborns are hepatosplenomegaly, meningoencephalitis, anemia and cardiac failure. Congenital transmission may cause abortion, premature birth, still birth and low body weight for the newborn [57].

The recommendation is that all newborns of women from an endemic area or with a previous diagnosis of Chagas disease should be investigated immediately after birth, when, theoretically, the parasitemia is high and more easily detected by the parasitological methods typically used in the acute phase of the infection, mainly microhematocrit, hemoculture of umbilical cord blood, placental histopathology (including immunohistochemistry) and PCR. In addition, serological testing should be performed, especially evaluating IgM antibodies. Accidents during birth delivery may contaminate the child with the mother's IgM. If the diagnosis is not conclusive, the child must be serologically examined six to nine months or later after birth, when the passive antibodies of the mother have disappeared. Even by this time, the success of etiological treatment is high and should be immediately administered after diagnosis confirmation [61]. If the congenital infection is not diagnosed, the child will likely receive a diagnosis some years later as a consequence of clinical disorders caused by the infection. Even in such a situation, the success of the etiological treatment is higher in children than in adults [38].

The diagnosis of congenital transmission may be performed by examination of the placenta. The placenta may be bigger than normal, pale, with edema, increased cotyledons and whitish in color. Histopathology and immunohistochemistry may detect parasites and/or parasite antigens. The basic lesion is a proliferation of Hofbauer cells, stromal infiltration by lymphocytes and histiocytes, edema, necrotic foci and vascular alterations. Parasites may also be detected in the Wharton gelatin of the umbilical cord.

Transplants: Transplants are complicated in both infection situations: when the donor is infected with *T. cruzi* or when the receptor of the organ is infected because the recipient of the transplant must use immunosuppressants to avoid organ rejection [62]. Thus, an acute phase or reagudization of the disease occurs in the first or second situation, respectively. Currently, the transplant recipient must be assisted by a team, including a parasitologist and immunologist, to perform the necessary laboratory evaluations during the first weeks after the transplant. The number of CD4 cells is important for monitoring the degree of immunosuppression (<200 µl of blood) and determining when the introduction of the etiological treatment for Chagas disease is necessary.

Laboratory accidents: Accidental infection may occur with people who work with the parasite in culture, animal models or with insects because all evolutionary forms of the parasite (except epimastigotes) are infectious when inoculated, ingested or in contact with mucous or skin lesions. Several cases of accidental infection were documented [63, 64] and some were fatal, as determined by the *T. cruzi* strain, inoculum and route of inoculation. The recommended prophylaxis measures are as follows: working with the parasite only after being well trained, using covered shoes and individual protection equipment (mask for eye and face protection, gloves), using alcohol to immediately clean the skin upon suspicion of contact with the parasite and always being attentive when working. It is advisable to perform serological tests of the personnel before they begin work with the parasite. This creates a baseline for the person before the exposition to the parasite, and the results can be compared later in the case of an accident.

Immunosuppressed patients: Immunosuppression can lead to chronic phase reactivation. This can occur due to the use of immunosuppression drugs, transplant-associated immunosuppression or immunosuppression associated with other diseases such as cancer or HIV/AIDS [62]. When intense, the immunosuppression causes disease reactivation due to cellular immune depression and symptoms, including myocarditis and meningoencephalitis. Neurological manifestations are the consequences of central nervous system

(CNS) lesions, including headache, fever, cognitive disturbances and seizures. The presence of tumor-like lesions is the most common event associated with the white matter [65].

Diagnostic confusion regarding tumor lesions with toxoplasmosis and neoplasms, such as CNS lymphoma, is common with magnetic resonance image (MRI). Meningoencephalitis may be confirmed with lumbar puncture of the cerebrospinal fluid (CSF), where the trypomastigote form of the parasite can be detected [65]. Patients with myocarditis present arrhythmias and refractory congestive heart failure followed by rapid fatal evolution. The diagnosis may be confirmed by epidemiological antecedents, dilated cardiomyopathy and conventional serological tests.

Immunosuppression (< 200 CD4+ cells/μl) may interfere with both parasitological and conventional serological tests because of changes in the parasitemia and antibody level. Parasites may be detected by fresh blood examination, microhematocrit, hemoculture, xenodiagnosis, in biopsy material, CSF [66] and PCR.

Final Considerations

As described, there are variable approaches to diagnosis. Currently, there are many available serological tests and more than that can be done, including improvement of antigens, which requires more precise knowledge of the etiological agent, reagents and techniques. The parasitological methods applicable for the majority of the cases are not used in clinical analysis laboratories and the more simple parasitological diagnostic methods are applicable only for the acute phase of the disease, a rare occurrence today in countries where the Chagas disease control programs are advanced. Even considering all the diagnostic possibilities, at least 2% of patients are not correctly diagnosed (false positive and false negative). There should be an emphasis on the discovery of rapid, simple and accurate tests that can utilize available fresh blood in endemic areas without the need of sophisticated equipment and specialized training.

References

[1] Romanã C. Acerca de um síntoma inicial de valor para el diagnóstico de forma aguda de la enfermedad de Chagas. La conjuntivitis esquizotripanósica unilateral. (Hipótesis sobre puerta de entrada conjuntival de la enfermedad). *Public MEPRA*. 1935; 22: 16-28.

[2] Mazza S, Freire RS. Manifestaciones cutáneas de inoculación, metastáticas y hematógenas en enfermedad de Chagas. Chagomas de inoculación, chagomas metastáticos y chagomas hematógenos. *Public MEPRA*. 1940; 46: 3-38.

[3] Brener Z. Therapeutic activity and criterion of cure on mice experimentally infected with *Trypanosoma cruzi*. *Rev. Inst. Med. Trop.* São Paulo. 1962; 4: 389-96.

[4] Camargo EP. Growth and differentiation in *Trypanosoma cruzi* I. Origin of metacyclic trypanosomes in liquid media. *Rev. Inst. Med. Trop.* São Paulo. 1964; 6: 93-100.

[5] Katzin A, Alves MJ, Abuin G, Colli W. Antigenuria in chronic chagasic patients detected by a monoclonal antibody raised against *Trypanosoma cruzi*. *Trans. R. Soc. Trop. Med. Hyg*. 1989; 83: 341-43.

[6] Lopes ER, Chapadeiro E, Batista SM, Cunha JG, Rocha A, Miziora L, Ribeiro JU, Patto RJ. Post-mortem diagnosis of chronic Chagas' disease: comparative evaluation of three serological tests on pericardial fluid. *Trans. R. Soc. Trop. Med. Hyg,* 1978; 72: 244-46.

[7] Sosa-Estani S, Segura EL. Etiological treatment in patients infected by *Trypanosoma cruzi*: experiences in Argentina. *Curr. Opin. Infect. Dis.* 2006; 19: 583-87.

[8] Luquetti AO, Tavares SBN, Oliveira RA, Siriano LR, Costa DG, Oliveira EC. Sorologia como critério de cura em pacientes tratados com benznidazol. Títulos obtidos em chagásicos não tratados por imunofluorecência indireta. *Rev. Soc. Bras. Med. Trop*, 2008; 41: 242-43.

[9] de Rezende JM, Moreira H. Chagasic megaesophagus and megacolon. Historical review and present concepts. *Arq. Gastroenterol*. 1988; 25: 32-43.

[10] Secretaria de Vigilância em Saúde do Ministério da Saúde. Consenso Brasileiro em Doença de Chagas. *Rev. Soc. Bras. Med. Trop.* 2005; 38 (Supl III).

[11] Brumpt E. Le xenodiagnostic. Application au diagnostic de quelques infections parasitaires et en particulier à la Trypanosomose de Chagas. *Bull. Soc. Pat. Exot.* 1914; 7: 706-10.

[12] Cerisola JÁ, Rohwedder R, Segura EL, Del Prado CE, Alvarez M, Martini GJW. El xenodiagnóstico. Buenos Aires. *Imp. Inst. Nac. Invest.* Cardiovasc., 1974; 157.

[13] dos Santos AH, da Silva IG, Rassi A. A comparative study between natural and artificial xenodiagnosis in chronic Chagas' disease patients. *Rev. Soc. Bras. Med. Trop.* 1995; 28: 367-73.

[14] de Lana M, da Silveira Pinto A, Barnabé C, Quesney V, Noel S, Tibayrenc M. *Trypanosoma cruzi*: compared vectorial transmissibility of three major clonal genotypes by *Triatoma infestans*. *Exp. Parasitol.* 1998; 90: 20-5.

[15] da Silveira Pinto A, de Lana M, Britto C, Bastrenta B, Tibayrenc M. Experimental *Trypanosoma cruzi* biclonal infection in *Triatoma infestans*: detection of distinct clonal genotypes using kinetoplast DNA probes. *Int. J. Parasitol.* 2000; 30: 843-48.

[16] Cedillos RA, Torrealba JW, Tonn RJ, Mosca W, Ortegón A. Artificial xenodiagnosis in Chagas disease. *Bol. Oficina Sanit. Panam.* 1982; 93: 240-49.

[17] Luz ZM, Coutinho MG, Cançado JR, Krettli AU. Hemoculture: sensitive technique in the detection of *Trypanosoma cruzi* in chagasic patients in the chronic phase of Chagas disease. *Rev. Soc. Bras. Med. Trop.* 1994; 27: 143-48.

[18] Castellani O, Ribeiro LV, Fernandes JF. Differentiation of *Trypanosoma cruzi* in culture *J. Protozool.* 1967; 14: 447-51.

[19] Avila HA, Sigman DS, Cohen LM, Millikan RC, Simpson L. Polymerase chain reaction amplification of *Trypanosoma cruzi* kinetoplast minicircle DNA isolated from whole blood lysates: diagnosis of chronic Chagas' disease. *Mol. Biochem. Parasitol.* 1991; 48: 211-21.

[20] Galvão LM, Chiari E, Macedo AM, Luquetti AO, Silva SA, Andrade AL. PCR assay for monitoring *Trypanosoma cruzi* parasitemia in childhood after specific chemotherapy. J. Clin. Microbiol. 2003; 41: 5066-70.

[21] Vergara U, Veloso C, Gonzalez A, Lorca M. Evaluation of an enzyme-linked immunosorbent assay for the diagnosis of Chagas' disease using synthetic peptides. *Am. J. Trop. Med. Hyg.* 1992; 46: 39-43.

[22] Umezawa ES, Nascimento MS, Kesper NJr, Coura JR, Borges-Pereira J, Junqueira AC, Camargo ME. Immunoblot assay using excreted-secreted

antigens of *Trypanosoma cruzi* in serodiagnosis of congenital, acute, and chronic Chagas' disease. *J. Clin. Microbiol.* 1996; 34: 2143-47.

[23] Toledo MJ, de Lana M, Carneiro CM, Bahia MT, Machado-Coelho GL, Veloso VM, Barnabé C, Tibayrenc M, Tafuri WL. Impact of *Trypanosoma cruzi* clonal evolution on its biological properties in mice. *Exp. Parasitol.* 2002; 100: 161-72.

[24] Macedo AM, Segato M. Implications of *Trypanosoma cruzi* intraspecific diversity in the pathogenesis of Chagas disease. In: Telleria J and Tibayrenc M. (Eds). American Trypanosomiasis Chagas Disease - One Hundred Years of Research. (1 ed, 489-522). London, England: *ELSEVIER.* 2010.

[25] Tibayrenc M, Brenière SF. *Trypanosoma cruzi*: major clones rather than principal zymodemes. *Mem. Inst. Oswaldo Cruz.* 1988; 83: 249-55.

[26] Saldaña A, Souza OE. *Trypanosoma rangeli*: epimastigote immunogenicity and cross-reaction with *Trypanosoma cruzi*. *J. Parasitol.* 1996; 82: 363-66.

[27] Santos LS, Torres RM, Machado-de-Assis GF, Bahia MT, Martins HR, Teixeira-Carvalho A, Coelho-dos-Reis JG, Albajar-Viñas P, Martins-Filho AO, de Lana M. In-house ELISA method to analyze anti-*Trypanosoma cruzi* IgG reactivity for differential diagnosis and evaluation of Chagas disease morbidity. *Rev. Soc. Bras. Med. Trop.* 2012; 45: 35-44.

[28] Vallejo GA, Guhl F, Chiari E, Macedo AM. Species specific detection of *Trypanosoma cruzi* and *Trypanosoma rangeli* in vector and mammalian hosts by polymerase chain reaction amplification of kinetoplast minicircle DNA. *Acta Trop.* 1999; 72: 203-12.

[29] Guerreiro C, Machado A. Da reação de Bordet e Gengou na moléstia de Carlos Chagas como elemento diagnóstico. *Brasil Med.* 1913; 27: 225-26.

[30] Camargo ME. Fluorescent antibody test for the serodiagnosis of American trypanosomiasis. Technical modification employing preserved culture forms of *Trypanosoma cruzi* in a slide test. *Rev. Inst. Med. Trop.* Sao Paulo. 1966; 8: 227-34.

[31] Ministério da Saúde. Resultado da avaliação dos kits para diagnóstico da doença de Chagas. Nota Técnica 03/06. 2006.

[32] Machado-Coelho GL, Vitor RW, Chiari CA, Antunes CM. Validity of serology for American trypanosomiasis with eluates from filter paper. *Mem. Inst. Oswaldo Cruz.* 1995; 90: 59-64.

[33] Umezawa ES, Silveira JF. Serological diagnosis of Chagas disease with purified and defined *Trypanosoma cruzi* antigens. *Mem. Inst. Oswaldo Cruz.* 1999; 94: 285-88.

[34] Ministério da Saúde, Coordenação de DST/AIDS e COSAH. Telelab Nº.11. Doença de Chagas - Triagem e diagnóstico sorológico em unidades hemoterápicas e laboratórios de saúde pública. *Brasília Manual,* 1998; 75.

[35] Krettli AU, Brener Z. Resistance against *Trypanosoma cruzi* associated to anti-living trypomastigote antibodies. *J. Immunol.* 1982; 128: 2009-12.

[36] Meira WS, Galvão LM, Gontijo ED, Machado-Coelho GL, Norris KA, Chiari E. *Trypanosoma cruzi* recombinant complement regulatory protein: a novel antigen for use in an enzyme-linked immunosorbent assay for diagnosis of Chagas' disease. *J. Clin. Microbiol.* 2002; 40: 3735-40.

[37] Luquetti AO, Ponce C, Ponce E, Esfandiari J, Schijman A, Revollo S, Añez N, Zingales B, Ramgel-Aldao R, Gonzalez A, Levin MJ, Umezawa ES, Franco da Silveira J. Chagas' disease diagnosis: a multicentric evaluation of Chagas Stat-Pak, a rapid immunochromatographic assay with recombinant proteins of *Trypanosoma cruzi. Diagn. Microbiol. Infect. Dis.* 2003; 46: 265-71.

[38] Coura JR, de Castro SL. A critical review on Chagas' disease chemotherapy. *Mem. Inst. Oswaldo Cruz.* 2002; 97: 3-24.

[39] Cançado JR. Long term evaluation of etiological treatment of Chagas disease with benznidazole. *Rev. Inst. Med. Trop.* São Paulo. 2002; 44: 29-37.

[40] Martins-Filho AO, Pereira ME, Carvalho JF, Cançado JR, Brener Z. Flow cytometry, a new approach to detect anti-live trypomastigote antibodies and monitor the efficacy of specific treatment in human Chagas' disease. *Clin. Diagn. Lab. Immunol.* 1995; 2: 569-73.

[41] Vitelli-Avelar DM, Sahtler-Avelar R, Wendling APB, Rocha RDR, Teixeira- Carvalho A, Martins NE, Dias JC, Rassi A, Luquetti AO, Elói-Santos SM, Martins-Filho OA. Non-conventional flow cytometry approaches to detect anti-*Trypanosoma cruzi* immunoglobulin G in clinical laboratory. *J. Immunol. Methods.* 2007; 318: 102-12.

[42] Krettli AU, Cançado JR, Brener Z. Effect of specific chemotherapy on the levels of lytic antibodies in Chagas's disease. *Trans. R. Soc. Trop. Med. Hyg.* 1982; 76: 334-40.

[43] Rassi A, Luquetti AO. Specific treatment for *Trypanosoma cruzi* infection (Chagas disease). In: Tyler KM and Miles MA. (Eds), *American trypanosomiasis*. (117-125). Boston, Kluwer Academic Publishers. 2003.

[44] Meira WS, Galvão LM, Gontijo ED, Machado-Coelho GL, Norris KA, Chiari E. Use of *Trypanosoma cruzi* recombinant complement regulatory protein to evaluate therapeutic efficacy following treatment of chronic chagasic patients. *J. Clin. Microbiol.* 2004; 42: 707-12.

[45] Krieger MA, Almeida E, Oelemann W, Lafaille JJ, Pereira JB, Krieger H, Carvalho MR, Goldenberg S. Use of recombinant antigens for the accurate immunodiagnosis of Chagas' disease. *Am. J. Trop. Med. Hyg.* 1992; 46: 427- 34.

[46] World Health Organization. Control of Chagas' disease report of a WHO Expert Committee. *World Health Organ. Tech. Rep.* 2002; Ser. 905.

[47] Rohwedder RW. Chagas' infection in blood donors and the possibility of its transmission by blood transfusion. *Bol. Chil. Parasitol.* 1969; 24: 88-93.

[48] Schmuñis GA. Epidemiology of Chagas disease in nonendemic countries: the role of international migration. *Mem. Inst. Oswaldo Cruz.* 2007; 107: 75-85.

[49] Goodman C, Chan S, Collins P, Haught R, Chen YJ. Ensuring blood safety and availability in the US: technological advances, costs, and challenges to payment. *Final report Transfusion.* 2003; 43: 3S-46S.

[50] Assal A, Aznar C. Chagas disease screening in the French blood donor population. Screening assays and donor selection. *Enf. Emerg.* 2007; 9: 38-40.

[51] Otani MM. Programa de avaliação externa para os testes de triagem sorológica de doadores de banco de sangue dos centros de referencia da America Latina: utilização de multipainel específico. Thesis, University of São Paulo. 2003.

[52] Saéz-Alquezar A, Otani MM, Sabino EC, Salles NA, Chamone DF. External serology quality control programs developed in Latin America with the support of PAHO from 1997 through 2000. *Rev. Panam. Salud. Publica.* 2003; 13: 91-102.

[53] Flores-Chávez M, Faez Y, Olalla JM, Cruz I, Gárate T, Rodríguez M, Blanc P, Cañavate C. Fatal congenital Chagas' disease in a non endemic area: a case report. *Cases J.* 2008: 1: 302.

[54] Bern C, Verastegui M, Gilman RH, Lafuente C, Galdos-Cardenas G, Calderon M, Pacori J, Del Carmen Abastoflor M, Aparicio H, Brady MF, Ferrufino L, Angulo N, Marcus S, Sterling C, Meguire JH. Congenital *Trypanosoma cruzi* transmission in Santa Cruz, Bolivia. *Clin. Infect. Dis.* 2009; 49: 1667-74.

[55] Brutus L, Castillo H, Bernal C, Salas NA, Schneider D, Santalla JA, Chipaux JP. Detectable *Trypanosoma cruzi* parasitemia during pregnancy and delivery as a risk factor for congenital Chagas disease. *Am. J. Trop. Med. Hyg.* 2010; 83: 1044-47.

[56] Apt W, Zulantay I, Solari A, Ortiz S, Oddo D, Corral G, Truyens C, Carlier Y. Vertical transmission of *Trypanosoma cruzi* in the Province of Choapa, IV Region, Chile. Preliminary report (2005-2008). *Biol. Res.* 2010; 43: 269-74.

[57] Carlier Y, Torrico F. Congenital infection with *Trypanosoma cruzi*: from mechanisms of transmission to strategies for diagnosis and control. *Rev. Soc. Bras. Med. Trop.* 2003; 36: 767-71.

[58] Luquetti AO, Passos AD, Silveira AC, Ferreira AW, Macedo V, Prata AR. The national survey of seroprevalence for evaluation of the control of Chagas disease in Brazil (2001-2008). *Rev. Soc. Bras. Med. Trop.* 2011; 44: 108-21.

[59] Burgos JM, Altcheh J, Bisio M, Duffy T, Valadares HM, Seidenstein ME, Piccinali R, Freitas JM, Levin MJ, Macchi L, Macedo AM, Freilij H, Schijman AG. Direct molecular profiling of minicircle signatures and lineages of *Trypanosoma cruzi* bloodstream populations causing congenital Chagas disease. *Int. J. Parasitol.* 2007; 37: 1319-27.

[60] Falla A, Herrera C, Fajardo A, Montilla M, Vallejo GA, Guhl F. Haplotype identification within *Trypanosoma cruzi* I in Colombian isolates from several reservoirs, vectors and humans. *Acta. Trop.* 2009; 110: 15-21.

[61] de Andrade A L, Zicker F, de Oliveira RM, Almeida Silva SAS, Luquetti A, Travassos LR, Almeida IC, de Andrade SS, de Andrade JG, Martelli CM. Randomised trial of efficacy of benznidazole in treatment of early *Trypanosoma cruzi* infection. *Lancet.* 1996; 348: 1407-13.

[62] Ferreira MS. Chagas disease and immunosupression. *Mem. Inst. Oswaldo Cruz.* 1999; 94: 325-27.

[63] Brener Z. Laboratory-acquired Chagas' disease: an endemic disease among parasitologists? In: Genes and Antigens of Parasites. A Laboratory Manual. Fundação Oswaldo Cruz. 1984; 3-9.

[64] Ministério da Saúde, Fundação Nacional da Saúde, Gerência Técnica de Doença de Chagas. Normas de segurança para infecções acidentais com o *Trypanosoma cruzi*, agente causador da doença de Chagas. *Rev. Patol. Trop.* 1997; 26: 129-30.

[65] Cordova E, Boschi A, Ambrosioni J, Cudos C, Corti M. Reactivation of Chagas' disease with central nervous system involvement in HIV-infected patients in Argentina, 1992-2007. *Int. J. Infect. Dis.* 2008; 12: 587-92.

[66] Sartori AM, Neto JE, Nunes EV, Braz LM, Caiaffa-Filho HH, Oliveira Oda C Jr, Neto VA, Shikanai-Yasuda MA. *Trypanosoma cruzi* parasitemia in chronic Chagas' disease: comparison between human immunodeficiency virus (HIV)-positive and HIV-negative patients. *J. Infect. Dis.* 2002; 186: 872-75.

In: Chagas Disease   ISBN: 978-1-62808-681-2
Editors: F. R. Gadelha, E.d.F. Peloso   © 2013 Nova Science Publishers, Inc.

Chapter VI

Chagas Disease Treatment

Eduardo de Figueiredo Peloso

Departamento de Bioquímica - Instituto de Biologia
Universidade Estadual de Campinas, Campinas-SP, Brazil

Abstract

Due to its clinical importance, patients diagnosed with Chagas disease should be treated as soon as possible. Although there is disagreement as to the percent cured through etiological treatment, depending on circumstances such as the stage of the disease, patient age and associated conditions, there is a consensus about its usefulness. Treatment is given in the acute and chronic phase, in cases of congenital infection, in cases of transplantation, in immunosuppressed patients and in cases of accidental infection. The drugs used for treatment are nifurtimox and benznidazole. Benznidazole is the only drug currently available in Brazil; nifurtimox is used in Central America but can be used as an alternative in cases of intolerance to benznidazole. Both are nearly 100% effective at curing patients of disease soon after infection. However, the effectiveness of both drugs decreases the longer the patient is infected. The advantages of the drugs used to prevent or delay the development of Chagas disease must be weighed against long-term treatment and possible adverse effects. After treatment, cure is confirmed via negative serology that is variable and depends on the stage of the disease. In the search for drugs with higher specificity and less collateral damage, some candidates (some with anti-fungal properties) have been noted, and others are already in clinical trials.

Introduction

Although the incidence and prevalence of Chagas disease has reduced considerably since the 1990s, the effect of human migration has led to the emergence of new cases in different countries where there are no vectors and the disease is not endemic [1].

The World Health Organization estimates that the morbidity and mortality combined account for an annual economic loss of more than US$ 6.5 billion in Latin America alone. However, despite the number of fatalities and the high cost associated with this disease, pharmaceutical companies have not shown a real interest in developing new drugs, leaving nifurtimox (NF) and benznidazole (BZ) as the first and only line of treatment for Chagas disease.

Nifurtimox and Benzonidazole

NF (4 [(5-nitrofurfurylidene) amino]-3-methylthiomorpholine-1,1-dioxide), is a nitrofuran derivative and BZ (N-benzyl-2-nitroimidazole-1-acetamide), a nitroimidazole derivative, that have been in use for almost 45 years [2]. Both nitroheterocyclic compounds are characterized by a nitro group linked to an aromatic ring [3] (Figure 1).

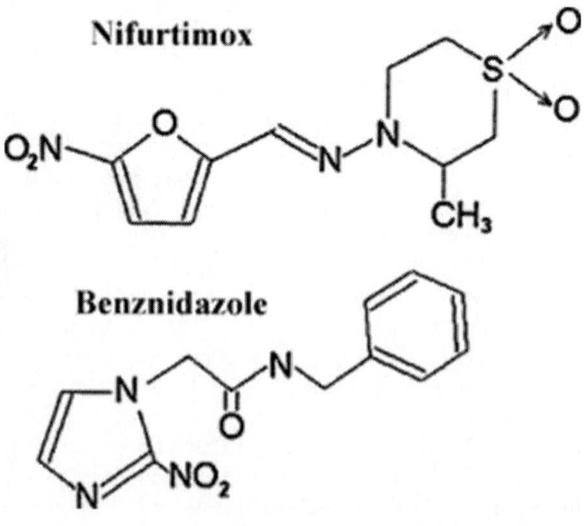

Figure 1. Chemical structure of nifurtimox and benzonidazole.

The use of both nifurtimox and benzonidaxole is strongly criticized due to their low effectiveness and severe side effects, especially in adults, resulting in 20 to 30% of patients discontinuing treatment [4]. The main side effects are anorexia, weight loss, alterations in mentation, excitability, sleepiness, gastrointestinal upset, such as nausea or vomiting, and occasionally intestinal colic and diarrhea. In the case of BZ, skin manifestations are the most notable (e.g., hypersensitivity and dermatitis with cutaneous eruptions). The main severe manifestations are bone marrow depression, thrombocytopenic purpura and agranulocytosis [5]. Toxicity studies with NF demonstrated neurotoxicity, testicular damage, ovarian toxicity, and deleterious effects in adrenal, colon, esophageal and mammary tissue. In the case of BZ, deleterious effects were observed in the adrenals, colon and esophagus. BZ also inhibits the metabolism of several xenobiotics biotransformed by the cytochrome P450 system. The reactive metabolites of BZ also react with fetal components *in vivo*. Both drugs exhibit significant mutagenic effects and were shown to be tumorigenic or carcinogenic in some studies.

Mechanism of Action of NF and BZ

Nifurtimox and benzonidazole function as prodrugs and therefore must undergo enzyme-mediated activation within the pathogen or the host to have cytotoxic effects.

The nitro group of both drugs is reduced by the action of nitroreductases (NTRs), inducing the formation of various free radical intermediates and nucleophilic metabolites. NTRs are divided into two groups based on oxygen sensitivity [6]. Type I NTRs are oxygen-insensitive, contain flavin mononucleotide (FMN) as a cofactor and function via a series of two-electron reductions of the conserved nitro group, leading to moieties that promote DNA damage.

This class of NTR is characteristically found within bacteria. The only trypanosomal enzyme shown to mediate this type of activity is prostaglandin F2α synthase (also known as "old yellow enzyme") [7], although only under anaerobic conditions.

Type II NTRs are ubiquitous, oxygen-sensitive, flavin adenine dinucleotide (FAD)- or FMN-containing enzymes that mediate a one-electron reduction of the nitro group generating an unstable nitro-radical. In the presence of oxygen, this radical undergoes futile redox cycling to produce superoxide (O_2^-) with the subsequent regeneration of the parent nitro-compound [6, 8].

Etiological Treatment of Chagas Disease

Considering the side effects of the two drugs used in the etiological treatment of Chagas disease, careful attention must be given to adequate dosing and management of adverse reactions that occur with varying severity in approximately 20% [9] or even 30-60% of patients treated in the chronic phase of the infection [10 - 11]. Additionally, the side effects of these drugs are well tolerated in infants [10, 12-14]. Thus, taking into account the possible adverse reactions associated with the use of drugs currently available, certain conditions must be taken into consideration, such as the stage of the disease, patient age and associated conditions, before starting etiological treatment of Chagas disease.

Stage of the Disease

Treatment in the Acute Phase

In the acute phase, defined as evidence of *T. cruzi* in direct examination of the peripheral blood, treatment should be performed in all cases and as fast as possible after diagnosis is confirmed.

However, treatment is not recommended during pregnancy due to drug toxicity [15]. Studies show that the use of NF and BZ is effective in the acute phase, achieving a cure rate above 80%. Antitrypanosomal treatment is recommended for all cases of acute and congenital Chagas disease, reactivated infection and infection in individuals younger than 18 years-old. Additionally, treatment can be initiated in adults aged 19 to 50 years without advanced heart disease, but treatment is considered optional in patients older than 50 years without advanced heart disease. Individualized treatment for adults should consider the potential benefit, duration of use and frequency of adverse side effects.

In addition, patients with human immunodeficiency or awaiting organ transplant, assessment of treatment criteria should be made with the objective of determining the most appropriate treatment [16].

Treatment of Congenital Infection

Congenital Chagas disease is considered an acute infection with compulsory notification. In addition to cases diagnosed by direct observation of the parasite, the majority of patients are identified by serology. Because maternal antibodies may persist in children up to 6 to 9 months after birth, as noted by serology, testing should be repeated after this period and, if positive, treatment should be initiated [15].

Treatment of the Chronic Infection

For children who recently entered the chronic phase of infection, the recommendations for treatment follow the same reasoning as described for acute infection. Thus, all children less than 12 years-old with positive serology should be treated. Although there is no evidence for the success of this therapy in adults in different circumstances, treatment can be initiated in those who recently entered the chronic phase of infection. For the purpose of treatment, a period of five to twelve years after the initial infection is considered "recent." For chronic infections of longer duration, treatment has been indicated for slight and digestive indeterminate and cardiac manifestations of disease. Following a significant amount of discussion regarding treatment in the chronic phase, a consensus was reached. It was agreed that it is best to treat all forms of infection, including cardiac and gastrointestinal, after examining each case individually and taking into account the risk-benefit ratio. As there is no evidence to supporting improved prognosis, treatment with BZ or NF should not be limited to patients affected by advanced cardiac and gastrointestinal manifestations of disease [15, 17]. However, from the perspective of public health programs, there is no indication for the large-scale treatment of adults in the chronic phase of infection. After 10-20 years of etiological treatment in the chronic phrase, patient serologies may become negative. Establishment of cure, especially in the chronic phase, depends on several factors: stage of disease, patient age, time course, parasitology and serology.

Treatment in the Case of Transplant

Due to the risk of transmission or reactivation of Chagas disease following organ transplantation, it is necessary to know if the donor or the recipient has positive serologies.For cases absolutely requiring organ transplantation between a serology-positive donor and serology-negative recipient, the donor must be treated with BZ, if possible, according to the standard treatment protocol for 60 days before transplantation. In any case, it is desirable to perform the transplantation before 10 to 14 days of etiological treatment. Regarding the recipient, the literature and experienced specialists suggest the following alternatives:

- Initiate treatment immediately after surgery, treating the patient initially for 10 days and performing serology on the 20th and 40th consecutive days. In the case of seroconversion, conventional therapy for the acute phase should be initiated;
- Undertake serial sampling and begin etiological treatment if acute infection is present.

If donor and recipient are positive, the infection should be considered chronic.

The recipient should be monitored and treatment should be initiated if reactivation occurs.

It is important to note that diagnosis in this situation requires detection of parasites in the patient's blood or tissues [15].

Treatment in Immunocompromised Patients

In immunocompromised patients, such as patients using immunosuppressants, patients with hematologic malignancies, or patients co-infected with human immunodeficiency virus, reactivation of Chagas disease can occur.

Reactivation of disease must be confirmed by direct visualization of parasites in peripheral blood, other fluids or organic tissues.

Following reactivation, treatment is indicated for a period of 60 days and may be extended up to 90 days depending on the patient's clinical condition. In patients without documented reactivation but with persistently high parasitemia, pre-symptomatic therapy has been proposed by some authors. However, there is the need for long follow-up periods for better evaluation of treatment efficacy [15].

Treatment of Accidental Infection

People who work with *T. cruzi* are considered infected when they accidentally break the skin during drill-cutting, have contact with mucous membranes, or encounter any other mechanism that enables the parasite to penetrate host physical barriers while handling material containing living parasites; live parasites can be present in samples for culture, vectors and laboratory infected animals, samples from patients suspected of high parasitemia and autopsy material. In the case of accidental infection, treatment (BZ, 7-10 mg/kg for ten days) is indicated immediately. Following the accidental exposure, blood parasitology and serology are performed for 10 to 15 days and serology is repeated 15, 30, and 60 days after exposure. Accidents with high parasite load should be treated for a minimum of 30 days. Accidentally infected individuals should undergo clinical and serological monitoring [15].

It is recommended that all laboratories that work with *T. cruzi* have NF or BZ available [15, 18] and should follow safety protocols. In case of an accident, the internal biosafety committee should be notified and procedures reevaluated.

It is noteworthy that in addition to NF or BZ, the specific treatment of cardiac or gastrointestinal manifestations is necessary.

Exceptions to Treatment

Due to the toxicity of NF and BZ, treatment should not be given to pregnant women, women of childbearing potential not using contraception or those who are lactating, people who ingest alcohol on a daily basis and individuals with hepatic or renal impairment. Treatment should not be prescribed in cases of co-infection with serious injuries associated with Chagas at any stage of the disease, except in cases of immunocompromised patients; reactivation of Chagas disease can occur resulting in the need for specific treatment [15].

Dose / Treatment

Despite the potential for cross-resistance, when monotherapy fails with one drug, the other can be used. In Brazil, BZ is the only drug currently

available, and if there is drug intolerance, NF may be used. Detailed dosing of
BZ and NF in the USA and Brazil are presented in the tables below:

**Table 1. Dosage of BZ and NF currently in use
in the United States of America**

Drug	Age group	Dosage and duration
Benznidazole	< 12 years	10mg/Kg per day orally in 2 divided doses for 60 days
	12 years or older	5-7mg/Kg per day orally in 2 divided doses for 60 days
Nifurtimox	≤ 10 years	15-20mg/Kg per day orally in 3 or 4 divided doses for 90 days
	11-16 years	12.5-15mg/Kg per day orally in 3 or 4 divided doses for 90 days
	17 years or older	8-10mg/Kg per day orally in 3 or 4 divided doses for 90 days

Source: Centers for Disease Control and Prevention - Evaluation and Treatment of
Chagas Disease in the United States: A Systematic Review – USA. Available in
http://www.cdc.gov/parasites/chagas/. Access made on 02/14/2013.

Table 2. Dosage of BZ and NF currently in use in Brazil

Drug	Age group	Dosage and duration
Benznidazole	Child	5-10mg/Kg per day orally in 2 or 3 divided doses for 60 days
	Adult	5mg/Kg per day orally in 2 or 3 divided doses for 60 days
Nifurtimox	Child	15mg/Kg per day orally in 3 divided doses for 60 to 90 days
	Adult	8-10mg/Kg per day orally in 3 divided doses for 60 to 90 days

Source: Ministério da Saúde/Brasil – Consenso Brasileiro em Doença de Chagas, 2005
[15].

It is important to consider that treatment failure can be accounted for not
only by the existence of strains of *T. cruzi* with natural drug resistance [19] but
also by a deficiency in the immune response [20]. According to Streiger and
colleagues [21], 95 children (aged 1-14 years) treated with BZ or NF in the

chronic phase of Chagas infection and followed for up to 24 years showed cure rates as high as 75% for children younger than 4 years old and 43% for children older than 9 years old. In another study, Fabro and colleagues [22] evaluated the efficacy of NF and/or BZ for 21 years in adults (17-46 years) in the chronic phase of Chagas disease. This study included 111 patients, 54 treated (27 with NF and 27 with BZ) and 57 untreated. According to the criteria of cure, the treatment was effective in 37% of patients and showed a protective effect in clinical outcomes.

Criteria of Cure

Negative serology has been considered the only method that demonstrates cure. Serological tests based on the investigation of the immune system response to the presence of the parasite or its antigens may remain positive for a long time even in the absence of *T. cruzi* [23].

Experts suggest that the time required for a patient's serology to become negative is variable and depends on the stage of the disease: 3-5 years in the acute phase, 1 year for congenital infections, 5-10 years for recent chronic phase and over 20 years in the chronic phase of long duration. In this phase, serology titers can either persist over 3 dilutions or demonstrate a progressive decline, which is suggestive of future negative serologies.

Serology techniques recommended include IIF, ELISA and indirect hemagglutination. All techniques are available on the market as diagnostic kits, and their implementation is relatively simple, with adequate sensitivity and specificity [24] when used in combination. These techniques allow a comparison between serum antibody titers before, during and after completion of treatment. In several countries, it has been shown that children below 12 years of age respond more quickly to treatment than adults. It is suggested, therefore, that serology follow up of treated patients should be performed for several years and that serology be done using different techniques and methodologies. The results should always be compared with the initial antibody levels. After 5 to 10 years of follow-up, if there are persistently positive serologies, it must be assumed that the treatment was ineffective [25]. Additionally, clinical evaluation of patients at least once a year is recommended. Clinical and complementary exams (chest X-ray, esophagus and colon, electrocardiogram (ECG), Holter, echocardiography) define the clinical form of the disease in seropositive patients [26].

At any moment in the evolution of the patient, the positive parasitology examinations indicate treatment failure [15]. Parasitology examinations should be performed before and after etiologic treatment and allow for the quantification of the patient parasitemia, which helps with clinical follow-up [25]. The parasitological tests used as criteria for cure include xenodiagnosis, blood culture and PCR [26]. The use of PCR for the detection of *T. cruzi* DNA or RNA to increase the diagnostic sensitivity of routinely used techniques has also been published in the literature. Comparative studies of samples from individuals with Chagas disease via parasitology, serology and molecular testing found that PCR was more sensitive than the other methods [27].

New Candidates for a Specific Treatment

Other drugs beside NF and BZ are being identified as new candidates for a more targeted treatment of Chagas disease.

T. cruzi requires endogenous steroids to proliferate and maintain cell viability. In experiments, fourth generation azole derivatives can induce in a radical parasitological cure of Chagas disease in acute and chronic phases. Such azoles include D0870 (Zeneca Pharmaceuticals, Macclesfield, UK) and SCH56592 (Posaconazole, Schering-Plough Research Institute, New Jersey, USA) with special pharmacokinetic properties and the ability to selectively inhibit the biosynthesis by the parasite of new steroids. These compounds were active against strains resistant to BZ and NF and kept their activity even in immunocompromised hosts [28]. Posaconazole that was recently registered in the European Union, Australia and the United States as a systemic antifungal is currently the strongest candidate for a new specific treatment for Chagas disease [29-30]. This drug is already registered for the treatment of invasive fungal infections and is currently undergoing Phase II clinical trials to evaluate its efficacy and safety for the specific treatment of chronic Chagas disease in humans [31].

TAK-187, an experimental antifungal triazole, was also investigated for its activity in the acute and chronic phases of Chagas disease in mice infected with *T. cruzi*. The results showed that TAK-187 administered orally at a dose of 20 mg/kg/day provided complete protection against mice mortality with high levels of parasitological cure (60% - 100%) regardless of the strain being targeted. TAK-187 is considered a potent anti-*T. cruzi* drug both *in vitro* and *in vivo*, even against strains resistant to nitrofuran and nitroimidazole. TAK-187 is also able to produce high levels of parasitological cure in models of acute and chronic phases of Chagas disease [32]. Further, it has been shown that TAK-187 is superior to BZ in preventing cardiac damage in murine models of Chagas disease [33].

Ravuconazole is another triazole with potent antifungal activity *in vitro* and *in vivo*, comparable or superior to other triazoles such as voriconazole and posaconazole. Ravuconazole at a dose of 15 mg/kg in experiments of acute infection caused by various strains of *T. cruzi* resistant to nitroimidazole and nitrofuran was able to induce parasitological cure in all animals infected with strain CL and in 58% of animals infected with strain Y; there was no cure in animals infected with the Colombian strain, however [34].

Another triazole, ketoconazole, suppressed parasitemia between animals infected with strains CL and Y. However, in mice infected with the Colombian strain and treated with triazole, parasitemia recurred in 35 days [32]. Further, it was shown that ketoconazole inhibits the growth of *T. cruzi in vitro* by blocking *de novo* biosynthesis of endogenous sterols, with inhibitory concentrations for amastigotes that are not toxic to host cells [35]. However, studies in a murine model and in humans have shown that ketoconazole is not effective in the chronic stage of the disease [35].

Allopurinol is a pyrazolopyrimidine used to treat gout. In the 1990s, its trypanocidal activity in mice and in cell cultures infected with *T. cruzi* was investigated. As results were similar to NF and BZ, with the advantage being lower toxicity, some researchers began to use it in humans. However, when used in doses of 300, 600 or 900 mg daily in the treatment of Chagas disease, two studies conducted in Bolivia and central Brazil found out that allopurinol was not effective at treating disease [36]. Since the introduction of BZ and NF, only allopurinol and a few azoles, such as itraconazole, fluconazole, and ketoconazole, have moved to clinical trials [37].

Megazol, a thiadizaole derivative, suppressed protein synthesis in amastigotes at concentrations lower than nitro-derivatives. Despite its noteworthy trypanocidal activity, megazol development was discontinued due to reports of *in vitro* mutagenic and genotoxic effects [38]. In an attempt to circumvent this undesired profile, megazol analogues were synthesized, but none have been found to be more potent than the prototype [39]. Although intense efforts have been directed to the identification of more active and less toxic megazol derivatives, the results are not encouraging [40].

Naphthoimidazoles, substances extracted from the tree of the genus Tabebuia, were quite effective against all forms of *T. cruzi* in mice. The toxicity of the compounds was decreased by making changes in the original molecule. Of the 60 naphthoimidazole derivatives, only 3 (N1, N2 and N3) were used.

The concentrations of the drugs required to inhibit 50% of parasites (IC_{50}) were almost equal to that of BZ; the only difference was in toxicity [41]. N1, N2 and N3 have low toxicities in mammalian cells, are active against all parasite forms, block the cell cycle, and lead to DNA fragmentation and morphological alterations in different organelles [42].

Mice infected with *T. cruzi* who developed chronic Chagas' disease decreased the number of inflammatory cells and fibrosis when treated with stem cells.

The transplantation of stem cells did not alter parasite burden, but there was compensation for damage caused during the years of aggression to the myocardium [43].

Finally, a very promising inhibitor of cruzain, the major cysteine protease in *T. cruzi*, is N-methyl-piperazine-urea-F-hF-vinyl-sulfone-phenyl (a.k.a. K777), which blocks the autocatalytic processing of the protein precursor of cruzain [44]. This drug is currently under an Investigational New Drug (IND) application to conduct studies [45]

Final Considerations

In the one hundred years since the first record describing the morphology and life cycle of *T. cruzi*, no vaccine or effective treatment for chronic cases has been developed [46].

In addition, the lack of interest from pharmaceutical companies and the absence of effective social policies in endemic states are responsible for the evolution of very limited pharmacotherapies.

Possible candidates are being considered and some are in clinical trials. In this sense, taking into account that NF and BZ are far from ideal trypanocidal drugs (e.g., very safe, very effective, very stable and inexpensive), the search continues for new compounds with anti-*T. cruzi* activity, with low toxicities and increased efficacies during the indeterminate and chronic phases. Thus, there is an urgent need to identify specific enzymes and metabolic pathways in the parasite that could be potential targets for drug development. Further, the parasite genome sequencing project, made available since 2005 [47], has opened the possibility of identifying new specific pathways and novel drug targets in the near future.

References

[1] Pérez-Molina JA, Pérez-Ayala A, Moreno S, Fernández-González MC, Zamora J, López-Velez R. Use of benznidazole to treat chronic Chagas' disease: a systematic review with a meta-analysis. *J. Antimicrob. Chemother.* 2009; 64: 1139-47.

[2] Salas CO, Faúndez M, Morello A, Maya JD, Tapia RA. Natural and Synthetic Naphthoquinones Active against *Trypanosoma Cruzi*: An Initial Step towards New Drugs for Chagas Disease. *Curr. Med. Chem.* 2011; 18: 144-61.

[3] Teixeira AR. Chagas disease. *Postgrad. Med. J.* 2006; 82: 788-98.

[4] Murta SM, Gazzinelli RT, Brener Z, Romanha AJ. Molecular characterization of susceptible and naturally resistant strains of *Trypanosoma cruzi* to benznidazole and nifurtimox. *Mol. Biochem. Parasitol.* 1998; 93: 203-14.

[5] Castro JA, de Mecca MM, Bartel LC. Toxic side effects of drugs used to treat Chagas' disease (American trypanosomiasis). *Hum. Exp. Toxicol.* 2006; 25: 471-79.

[6] Wilkinson SR, Taylor MC, Horn D, Kelly JM, Cheeseman I. A mechanism for cross-resistance to nifurtimox and benznidazole in trypanosomes. *Proc. Natl. Acad. Sci. USA.* 2008; 105: 5022-27.

[7] Kubata BK, Kabututu Z, Nozaki T, Munday CJ, Fukuzumi S, Ohkubo K, Lazarus M, Maruyama T, Martin SK, Duszenko M, Urade Y. A key role for old yellow enzyme in the metabolism of drugs by *Trypanosoma cruzi. J. Exp. Med.* 2002; 196: 1241-51.

[8] Wilkinson SR, Bot C, Kelly JM, Hall BS. Trypanocidal Activity of Nitroaromatic Prodrugs: Current Treatments and Future Perspectives. *Curr. Topics in Med. Chem.* 2011; 11: 2072-84.

[9] Viotti R, Vigliano C, Armenti H, Segura E. Treatment of chronic Chagas disease with benznidazole: clinical and serologic evolution of patients with long term follow-up. *Am. Heart J.* 1994; 127: 151-162.

[10] Cançado JR. Long term evaluation of etiological treatment of Chagas disease with benzonidazole. *Rev. Inst. Med. Trop. São Paulo.* 2002; 44: 1-20.

[11] Carpintero DJ. Uso del ácido tióctico para La prevención de los efectos secundarios provocados por el benznidazol en pacientes con infección de Chagas crónica. *Medicina* (Buenos Aires). 1983; 43: 285-90.

[12] Sosa ES. Tratamiento de la enfermedad de Chagas con benznidazol y acido tióctico. *Medicina.* 2004; 64: 1-6.

[13] Freilij H, Altcheh J. Respuesta terapéutica al nifurtimox en pacientes de edad pediátrica com enfermedad de Chagas cronica de la ciudad de Buenos Aires, Argentina. *Rev. Patol. Trop.* 1998; 27 (Supl): 17-9.

[14] De Andrade AL, Zicker F, de Oliveira RM, Almeida Silva S, Luquetti A, Travassos LR, Almeida IC, de Andrade SS, de Andrade JG, Martelli CM. Randomised trial of efficacy of benzonidazole in treatment of early *Trypanosoma cruzi* infection. *Lancet.* 1996; 348: 1407- 13.

[15] Secretaria de Vigilância em Saúde do Ministério da Saúde. Consenso Brasileiro em Doença de Chagas. *Rev. Soc. Bras Med. Trop.* 2005; 38 (Supl III).

[16] Bern C, Montgomery SP, Herwaldt BL, Rassi A Jr, Marin-Neto JA, Dantas RO, Maguire JH, Acquatella H, Morillo C, Kirchhoff LV, Gilman RH, Reyes PA,Salvatella R, Moore AC. Evaluation and treatment of Chagas disease in the United States: a systematic review. *JAMA.* 2007; 298: 2171-81.

[17] Cançado JR. Quimioterapia da doença de Chagas: uma visão atual. Tópicos em Gastroenterologia (2ª edition). Rio de Janeiro, Brazil: Medsi. 1991.

[18] Coura JR, Castro SL. A critical review on Chagas' disease chemotherapy. *Mem. Inst. Oswaldo Cruz.* 2002; 97: 3-24.

[19] Braga MS, Lauria-Pires L, Argañaraz ER, Nascimento RJ, Teixeira AR. Persistent infections in chronic Chagas' disease patients treated with anti-*Trypanosoma cruzi* nitroderivatives. *Rev. Inst. Med. Trop.* São Paulo. 2000; 42: 157-61.

[20] Ferraz ML, Gazzinelli RT, Alves RO, Urbina JA, Romanha AJ. The Anti-*Trypanosoma cruzi* activity of posaconazole in a murine model of acute Chagas' disease is less dependent on gamma interferon than that of benznidazole. *Antimicrob Agents Chemother.* 2007; 51: 1359-64.

[21] Streiger ML, del Barco ML, Fabbro DL, Arias ED, Amicone NA. Estudo longitudinal e quimioterapia específica em crianças, com doença de Chagas crônica, residentes em área de baixa endemicidade da República Argentina. *Rev. Soc Bras Med. Trop.* 2004; 37: 365-75.

[22] Fabbro DL, Streiger ML, Arias ED, Bizai ML, del Barco M, Amicone NA. Trypanocide treatment among adults with chronic Chagas disease living in Santa Fe city (Argentina), over a mean follow-up of 21 years: parasitological, serological and clinical evolution. *Rev. Soc. Bras. Med. Trop.* 2007; 40: 1-10.

[23] Rassi A, Amato Neto V, de Siqueira AF, Ferriolli Filho F, Amato VS, Rassi GG, Rassi Junior A. Tratamento da fase crônica da doença de

Chagas com nifurtimox associado a corticóide. *Rev. Soc. Bras. Med. Trop.* 2002; 35: 547-50.

[24] Zicker F, Smith PG, Luquetti AO, Oliveira OS. Mass screening for *Trypanosoma cruzi* infections using the imunofluorescence, ELISA and haemagglutination tests on serum samples and on blood eluates from filter–paper. *Bull World Health Org.* 1990; 68: 465-71.

[25] Silveira CA, Castillo E, Castro C. Avaliação do tratamento específico para o *Trypanosoma cruzi* em crianças, na evolução da fase indeterminada. *Rev. Soc. Bras. Med. Trop.* 2000; 33: 191-96.

[26] Cançado JR. Tratamiento específico da doença de Chagas crônica pelo Benznidazol. *Rev. Patol. Trop.* 1998; 27: 21-3.

[27] Jackson Y, Chatelain E, Mauris A, Holst M, Miao Q, Chappuis F, Ndao M. Serological and parasitological response in chronic Chagas patients 3 years after nifurtimox treatment. *BMC Infect. Dis.* 2013; 13:13:85.

[28] Urbina JA. Chemotherapy of Chagas disease. *Curr. Pharm. Dis.* 2002; 9: 287-95.

[29] Urbina JA, Payares G, Contreras LM, Liendo A, Sanoja C, Molina J, Piras M, Piras R, Perez N, Wincker P, Loebenberg D. Antiproliferative effects and mechanism of action of SCH 56592 against *Trypanosoma (Schizotrypanum) cruzi: in vitro* and *in vivo* studies. *Antimicrob. Agents Chemother.* 1998; 42: 1771-77.

[30] Molina J, Martins-Filho O, Brener Z, Romanha AJ, Loebenberg D, Urbina JA. Activities of the triazole derivate SCH 56592 (Posaconazole) against drug-resistant strains of the protozoan parasite *Trypanosoma* (Schizotrypanum) *cruzi* in immunocompetent and immunosuppressed murine host. *Antim. Agents Chemoth.* 2000; 44: 150-55.

[31] Urbina JA. New insights in Chagas disease treatment. *Drugs Fut.* 2010; 35:409-19.

[32] Urbina JA, Payares G, Sanoja C, Molina J, Lira R, Brener Z, Romanha AJ. Parasitological cure of acute and chronic experimental Chagas disease using the long- acting experimental triazole TAK-187. Activity against drug-resistant *Trypanosoma cruzi* strains. *Intern. J. Antimicrobial. Agents.* 2003; 21: 39-48.

[33] Corrales M, Cardozo R, Segura MA, Urbina JÁ, Basombrio MA. Comparative efficacies of TAK-187, a long-lasting ergosterol biosynthesis inhibitor, and benznidazole in preventing cardiac damage in a murine model of Chagas' disease. *Antimicrob Agents Chemother.*2005; 49: 1556-60.

[34] Diniz LF, Caldas IS, Guedes PMM, Crepalde G, de Lana M, Carneiro CM, Talvani A, Urbina JA, Bahia MT. Effects of Ravuconazole Treatment on Parasite Load and Immune Response in Dogs Experimentally Infected with *Trypanosoma cruzi*. *Antimicrob. Agents Chemother*. 2010; 54: 2979-86.

[35] Buckner FS. Sterol 14-demethylase inhibitors for *Trypanosoma cruzi* infections. *Adv. Exp. Med. Biol*. 2008; 625: 61-80.

[36] Rassi A, Luquetti AO, Rassi A Jr, Rassi GG, Rassi SG, DA Silva IG, Rassi AG. Specific treatment for *Trypanosoma cruzi*: lack of efficacy of allopurinol in the human chronic phase of Chagas disease. *Am. J. Trop. Med. Hyg*. 2007; 76: 58-61.

[37] de Castro SL, Batista DGJ, Batista MM, BatistaW, Daliry A, de Souza EM, Menna-Barreto RFS, Oliveira GM, Salomão K, Silva CF, Silva PB, Nazaré M, Soeiro C. Experimental Chemotherapy for Chagas Disease: AMorphological, Biochemical, and Proteomic Overview of Potential *Trypanosoma cruzi* Targets of Amidines Derivatives and Naphthoquinones. *Mol. Biol. International*. 2011; 2011.

[38] Nesslany F, Brugier S, Mouries MA, Curieux FL, Marzin D. *In vitro* and *in vivo* chromosomal aberrations induced by megazol. *Mut. Res*. 2004; 560:147–58.

[39] Carvalho AS, Menna-Barreto RFS, Romeiro NC, De Castro SL, Boechat N. Design, synthesis and activity against *Trypanosoma cruzi* of azaheterocyclic analogues of megazol. *Med. Chem*. 2007; 3: 460-65.

[40] de Souza KSEM, Carvalho SA, da Silva EF, Fraga CAM, Barbosa HS, de Castro SL. *In Vitro* and *In Vivo* Activities of 1,3,4-Thiadiazole-2-Arylhydrazone Derivatives of Megazol against *Trypanosoma cruzi*. *Antimicrob. Agents Chemother*. 2010; 54: 2023-31.

[41] Furtado F. Dobradinha contra Chagas. Ciência Hoje. 2006; 39: 44-5.

[42] Menna-Barreto RFS, Corrêa JR, Cascabulho CM, Fernandes MC, Pinto AV, Soares MJ, et al. Naphthoimidazoles promote different death phenotypes in *Trypanosoma cruzi*. *Parasitol*. 2009; 136:1-12.

[43] dos Santos RR, Soares MB, de Carvalho AC. Transplante de células da medula óssea no tratamento da cardiopatia chagásica crônica. *Rev. Soc. Bras. Med. Trop*. 2004; 37: 490-95.

[44] Engel JC, Doyle PS, Hsieh I, McKerrow JH. Cysteine protease inhibitors cure an experimental *Trypanosoma cruzi* infection. *J. Exp. Med*. 1998; 188: 725-34.

[45] Sajid M, Robertson SA, Brinen LS, McKerrow JH. Cruzain: the path from target validation to the clinic. *Adv. Exp. Med. Biol.* 2011; 712: 100-15.

[46] Bestetti RB, Martins CA, Cardinalli-Neto A. Justice where justice is due: A posthumous Nobel Prize to Carlos Chagas (1879-1934), the discoverer of American Trypanosomiasis (Chagas´disease). *Int. J. Cardiology.* 2009; 134: 9-16.

[47] El-Sayed NM, Myler PJ, Bartholomeu DC, Nilsson D, Aggarwal G, Tran AN, Ghedin E, Worthey EA, Delcher AL, Blandin G, Westenberger SJ, Caler E, Cerqueira GC, Branche C, Haas B, Anupama A, Arner E, Aslund L, Attipoe P, Bontempi E, Bringaud F, Burton P, Cadag E, Campbell DA, Carrington M, Crabtree J, Darban H, da Silveira JF, de Jong P, Edwards K, Englund PT, Fazelina G, Feldblyum T, Ferella M, Frasch AC, Gull K, Horn D, Hou L, Huang Y, Kindlund E, Klingbeil M, Kluge S, Koo H, Lacerda D, Levin MJ, Lorenzi H, Louie T, Machado CR, McCulloch R, McKenna A, Mizuno Y, Mottram JC, Nelson S, Ochaya S, Osoegawa K, Pai G, Parsons M, Pentony M, Pettersson U, Pop M, Ramirez JL, Rinta J, Robertson L, Salzberg SL, Sanchez DO, Seyler A, Sharma R, Shetty J, Simpson AJ, Sisk E, Tammi MT, Tarleton R, Teixeira S, Van Aken S, Vogt C, Ward PN, Wickstead B, Wortman J, White O, Fraser CM, Stuart KD, Andersson B. The genome sequence of *Trypanosoma cruzi*, etiologic agent of Chagas disease. *Science.* 2005; 309: 409-15.

In: Chagas Disease ISBN: 978-1-62808-681-2
Editors: F. R. Gadelha, E.d.F. Peloso © 2013 Nova Science Publishers, Inc.

Chapter VII

New Targets for the Development of an Improved Therapy for Chagas Disease

Eduardo de Figueiredo Peloso
and Fernanda Ramos Gadelha
Departamento de Bioquímica, Instituto de Biologia
Universidade Estadual de Campinas, Campinas-SP, Brazil

Abstract

Improved therapeutic agents against Chagas disease with higher efficacy and lower toxicity are urgently needed. The drugs presently used in treatment were discovered empirically, but current rational drug design offers a new approach that can make this search more pragmatic. A better understanding of the biology of *T. cruzi* will help identify unique and relevant targets for the development of a more specific therapy and will therefore lead to one that is more effective and less toxic to the vertebrate host. This chapter outlines the current understanding of the criteria for the development of an appropriate anti-trypanosoma drug and highlights the unique molecules involved in important pathways of parasite metabolism that have been noted as possible therapeutic targets. Among the most promising ones mentioned here are inhibitors of *T. cruzi* carbohydrate metabolism; ergosterol biosynthesis; calcium homeostasis; cruzain, the main cysteine protease of the parasite; polyamine homeostasis; protein tyrosine phosphatases; trans-sialidase; and the proteins related to the trypanothione network. The contribution of each one of these molecules to the survival of *T. cruzi*, and in some cases, its virulence and infectivity, will be addressed. Additionally, the reason these molecules are selected as potential targets for drug development and their available inhibitors, if any, will be discussed.

Introduction

Over the last few decades, considerable efforts have been made to control the transmission of *Trypanosoma cruzi*. In the absence of a safe and efficient vaccine [1], chemotherapy together with vector control is the most significant strategy to control the spread of this disease. The current chemotherapy in use was derived empirically many decades ago [2], and unfortunately, as described in Chapter VI, is unsatisfactory in terms of safety and efficacy. Further, resistance to commonly used insecticides to control insect vectors is also a concern [3].

Drug discovery in trypanosomatids has been achieved mainly through the screening of known compounds for activity against whole parasites. Another approach is screening compounds against defined molecular targets, known in the last few decades as "rational drug design" [4]. Several criteria should be met to develop appropriate drugs [5], and in the case of trypanosomes, these include selectivity (i.e., the desired target is not present or it is distinct from those in the host); "drugability" (the target molecule has a small molecule-binding pocket); appropriate biochemical properties (the target has a low turnover rate and/or catalyzes a bottleneck step within a pathway); validation (the target is essential for parasite proliferation and survival); "assayability" (specific, inexpensive and high-throughput screens are available using target compounds expressed *in vitro*); and low potential for the development of drug resistance [4]. In addition to that, the targets should not be strain-restricted to ensure their applicability in different endemic regions and, above all, the lack or low degree of toxicity is essential.

Taking all this into consideration, biochemical pathways common to trypanosomatids but absent from the mammalian host have long been regarded as potential drug targets. Genome sequencing of *T. cruzi* [6], as well as the advances in proteomics, biochemistry and in understanding parasite cell biology, has provided a framework for comparative biochemistry between parasite and mammalian hosts in the quest for drug targets [6]. Herein, some potential ones will be addressed and their relevance for *T. cruzi* survival will be highlighted.

Carbohydrate Metabolism

Glycolysis is considered a promising target for the development of a new therapy because it not only has an important role in ATP production but also has unique features in trypanosomes. In other eukaryotic cells, such as in the mammalian host, all of the glycolytic enzymes are present in the cytosol; however, in the kinetoplastids the first seven enzymes of glycolysis are localized to the glycosome [reviewed in 7]. Another important pathway for glucose utilization is the pentose phosphate pathway (PPP), which maintains a pool of the NADPH + H$^+$ that is necessary for reducing power for biosynthetic reactions and in the defense against oxidative stress, and it is involved in the generation of ribose 5P, which is employed in nucleotide synthesis. Apart from its cytosolic localization, the PPP is also believed to be present, at least in part, in the glycosome [8, reviewed in 7]. Once these enzymes are present inside an organelle, many regulatory mechanisms that exist in other eukaryotic cells do not function in trypanosomes [9]; for instance, hexokinase and phosphofructokinase, key regulatory enzymes in most glycolytic systems, are little or not at all affected by most common effectors [9].

Theoretical calculations and gene knockout experiments have demonstrated that glycolysis constitutes a valid drug target. Substantial work has attempted to elucidate the structure/kinetic parameters of glycolytic and PPP enzymes, such as glyceraldehyde-3-phosphate dehydrogenase, hexokinase and glucose-6-phosphate dehydrogenase. This work has led to the design of very potent inhibitors that were also effective on other trypanosomatids. In this sense, due to structural differences compared with their mammalian counterparts [9, reviewed in 7], the enzymes from glycolysis and PPP have been considered good targets for drug development.

Sterol Biosynthesis

T. cruzi, such as most fungi and yeasts, requires specific sterols for cell viability and proliferation in all stages of its life cycle [10]. Trypanosomatids contain sterols in the inner mitochondrial, glycosomal and plasma membranes that are involved in membrane fluidity and permeability, modulation of activity of membrane-bound proteins and ion channels [11]. Sterol biosynthesis enzymes have been found in the endoplasmic reticulum, mitochondrion and glycosomes, implying that there are multiple regulatory functions of endogenous sterols in trypanosomatids [11]. Unlike the human host, the main sterol in *T. cruzi* is ergosterol instead of cholesterol, turning the ergosterol biosynthesis pathway into a promising target for anti-trypanosomal chemotherapy [11]. Among the enzymes of this pathway, some have been spotted as good targets, such as HMG-CoA reductase (inhibited by statins used in humans for the reduction of cholesterol levels), farnesyl diphosphate synthase (target for bisphosphonates, used in humans as an antiosteoporosis drug) [12], squalene synthase (inhibited by quinuclidine derivatives) [13], sterol 24-methyl transferase (not present in humans and its inhibition by azasterols is highly selective) [14] and sterol 14α-demethylsae.

Sterol 14α-demethylase has the advantage over the others because its inhibitors, imidazole and triazole derivatives, are already efficiently used as antifungal agents in clinical medicine and in agriculture [15]. Inhibitors of this enzyme obtained from antifungal drug development programs can be used in anti-trypanosomal chemotherapy almost immediately. Combining imidazole and triazole derivatives with the currently available clinical antiprotozoan drugs should allow for decreases in drug dosages, thus minimizing their side effects and toxicity and shortening treatment time [11].

Calcium Homeostasis

Calcium plays an important role in cell signaling. Consequently, its intracellular levels have to be extremely regulated. In eukaryotic cells, transient changes in intracellular concentrations of Ca^{2+} have been associated with gene transcription, cell cycle regulation and cell proliferation. Disruption of calcium homeostasis usually induces cell damage, leading to cell death by apoptosis or necrosis [16].

In *T. cruzi*, the plasma membrane, mitochondrion and endoplasmic reticulum transporters and channels are involved in Ca^{2+} homeostasis. The acidocalcisomes have an important role in calcium and pH homeostasis as they are the primary reservoir of Ca^{2+} in these parasites [reviewed in 17].

Various studies have demonstrated the crucial role of Ca^{2+} as a second messenger in distinct pathways and in different trypanosomatids, e.g., as variant surface glycoprotein release in *Trypanosoma brucei* [18], stimulating an adenylyl cyclase [19] and a cAMP phosphodiesterase in *T. cruzi* [20], involved in *T. brucei* cellular differentiation [21] and in *Leishmania major*, where the Ca^{2+} influx and activation of calcineurin signaling is required for *L. major* differentiation and adaptation to cellular stress faced during infection of the mammalian host [22]. Most importantly, calcium plays an important role in cell invasion; in *T. cruzi* trypomastigotes, the cytoplasmic Ca^{2+} concentration increases during interaction with host cells [23], and in *Leishmania mexicana amazonensis*, a correlation has been established between Ca^{2+} signaling during invasion and virulence [24]. All these data reinforce the role of Ca^{2+} in parasite survival and note that calcium homeostasis is an important therapeutic target, not only in *T. cruzi* but also in other trypanosomatids.

In addition to that, calmodulin (CaM), the ubiquitous intracellular calcium-binding regulator, maintains 99% of its amino acid sequence between distinct trypanosomatids and 89% of its amino acid sequence between *T. cruzi* and vertebrate CaM. Once relevant biochemical differences between *T. cruzi* CaM and vertebrates were found, this protein was seen as an excellent target for chemotherapies [reviewed in 17].

Cysteine Protease

Proteases or proteinases are enzymes that break peptide bonds between amino acids in proteins, leading to the activation or inactivation of different enzymes. The cysteine protease requires a cysteine residue in the active site for hydrolysis and has been detected in a variety of organisms. They have been implicated in many processes related to parasite life cycle and pathogenesis [25], making them suitable targets for the design of specific inhibitors.

In *T. cruzi*, the major proteolytic activity of all stages of the life cycle is due to the presence of cruzipain (a.k.a, cruzain (a recombinant protein) or G57/51) [26]. Interestingly, depending on the life cycle stage in *T. cruzi*, cruzain has different intracellular locations; it is found on the cell surface of amastigotes or in the endosomal/lysosomal compartment of epimastigotes [27].

Cruzain is involved in many biological roles: immune evasion, where it prevents macrophage activation allowing *T. cruzi* survival and proliferation and in this way favoring the spread of infection [25, 28]; cell remodeling during the metacyclogenesis process [29]; mediating anti-apoptotic mechanisms in *T. cruzi* infected myocardium *in vitro* [30]; and many others.

Interestingly, aside from protease sequence alterations, a lower cruzain activity was observed when attenuated strains were compared to virulent ones [31].

The analogous cysteine proteinase target in *T. brucei*, brucipain, and cruzain, share significant homology (59%) in amino acid sequences, and when compared to mammalian proteinases, are most related to cathepsin L (~45%) [26]. Cruzain has been crystallized and exploited for the rational design of synthetic proteinase inhibitors [26]. In this sense, by blocking the autocatalytic processing of cruzain precursor protein, "chemical knockout" with cysteine protease inhibitors was lethal to *T. cruzi* with negligible mammalian toxicity [32], and as described in Chapter VI, one of these inhibitors (K777) is being considered as a therapeutic candidate by the National Institute of Health (NIH) [33].

Polyamine Homeostasis

Polyamines are a group of organic compounds containing two or more amino groups and are present in most eukaryotic cells. Polyamines, e.g., putrescine, and their derivatives, e.g., spermine or spermidine, are involved in a variety of relevant functions essential to macromolecular synthesis, cell survival, proliferation and differentiation [34-36]. Interestingly, their concentration and the activity of their biosynthetic enzymes are increased in cells with a high proliferation rate, such as cancerous cells and parasitic organism [reviewed in 37].

T. cruzi has a distinct polyamine metabolism when compared to the mammalian host and other trypanosomatids [38]. Most importantly, spermidine plays a relevant role in these organisms because it is the precursor of N^1, N^8-bis-glutathionyl-spermidine (trypanothione), a dithiol unique to trypanosomatids and fundamental for reactive oxygen species (ROS) detoxification, which will be discussed below.

Due to the relevance of polyamine biosynthesis, the inhibition of its biosynthetic pathway has been successfully applied to treat the Sleeping sickness, caused by *T. brucei*, and has opened the possibility that polyamine homeostasis may also be an important drug target in other trypanosomatids of human importance, such as *T. cruzi* and *Leishmania* spp [reviewed in 37].

Although it does not have a complete polyamine biosynthetic pathway, *T. cruzi* express both AdoMet decarboxylase (AdoMetDC) and spermidine synthase. In *T. cruzi*, ornithine decarboxylase (ODC), the first enzyme of this pathway, has not been identified, and the parasites rely on the uptake of exogenous putrescine; once putrescine is transported into the cell, it can be converted into spermidine (and spermine) [37, 38]. *T. cruzi* enzymes involved in polyamines biosynthesis are distinct to those in the mammalian host. In this sense, the primary structure of *T. cruzi* AdoMetDC has important differences compared to that of the mammalian enzyme [34]. MDL73811, an AdoMetDC inhibitor, decreased the capacity of *T. cruzi* to infect and multiply in rat heart myoblast [39].

In addition to inhibiting the enzymes of the polyamine biosynthetic pathway, other potential targets are using polyamine analogues to interfere with polyamine function and polyamine transport [reviewed in 37].

Protein Tyrosine Phosphatase

Phosphorylation and dephosphorylation via protein kinases and phosphatases, respectively, end up being important post-translational modifications. The most predominant phosphorylation sites in eukaryotic cells are in serine, threonine and tyrosine residues in proteins [40]. The phosphorylation status of proteins can regulate many signaling processes, such as cell cycle, differentiation, metabolism and other biological pathways [41]. Therefore, the pharmacological targeting of phosphatases involved in these processes can be an effective therapeutic strategy.

In relation to trypanosomatid protein phosphatases, various parasite-specific protein phosphatases have been identified. However, their molecular functions and the signaling pathways in which they are involved are not well understood [42]. Comparison of kinetoplastid phosphatomes revealed interesting differences; *T. brucei* has a unique and smaller phosphatome than *T. cruzi* and *Leishmania* spp [40]. As kinetoplastid phosphatase genes have low similarity to their vertebrate counterparts, targeting essential protein phosphatases may be an important strategy in the development of a more specific therapy to treat Chagas disease [40].

Among *T. cruzi* protein phosphatases, two protein tyrosine phosphatases (TcPTP1 and TcPTP2) were identified in the *T. cruzi* genome [43] with 15% homology with a human protein tyrosine phosphatase (PTP1B) [44] and were noted as possible drug targets. Interestingly, TcPTP1 was inhibited by 3-(3,5-dibromo-4-hydroxy-benzoyl) - 2 - ethyl - benzofuran - 6 - sulfonic acid- (4-(thiazol-2-ylsulfamyl) -phenyl)-amide (BZ3), a PTP1B inhibitor [45]. *T. cruzi* trypomastigote treated with BZ3 had decreased infectivity compared to untreated cells, raising the possibility that phosphorylation and dephosphorylating events take place in many events of parasite-host cell interaction. Additionally, metacyclogenesis induced by nutritional stress was accelerated in the presence of BZ3 [45]. Due to the high degree of homology between TcPTP2 and TcPTP1 (97%) [46], this effect could also be a result of TcPTP2 inhibition [45]. Future experiments to validate TcPTP1 as a potential therapeutic target are still needed, and inhibition of TcPTP2 activity should also be beneficial from a therapeutic standpoint [46].

Trans-Sialidase

Sialic acids, the generic term for the *N*- or *O*-substituted derivatives of neuraminic acid, are crucial for *T. cruzi* survival in the mammalian host [47, 48]. Because *T. cruzi* cannot synthesize sialic acid, this carbohydrate is acquired from host glycoconjugates through a glycosyl-transfer, mainly to parasite mucins, catalyzed by trans-sialidase (TS) [47, 49], thereby allowing parasite evasion from the immune system [48]. In *T. cruzi*, TS activity has also been related to recognition, host cell attachment and invasion [47], protection of epimastigotes from the glycolytic enzymes present in the gut of the insect vector [50], and trypomastigote escape from the parasitophorous vacuole [51]. Interestingly, *T. brucei* do not express TS in bloodstream forms, while *T. cruzi* has increased expression in these forms when compared to the epimastigote form (17%) [52]. In epimastigotes, TS is expressed in the stationary phase of growth and is structurally different from the trypomastigote enzyme [53].

Considering the specific need of *T. cruzi* to obtain sialic acid through TS-mediated transfers from host sources, the absence of this enzyme in the vertebrate host, the lack of alternatives to this pathway in the parasite and other TS distinct roles in the pathogenesis of Chagas disease, this enzyme serves as a potential drug target [reviewed in 54].

Several attempts to obtain suitable *T. cruzi* TS inhibitors have been made, especially once its 3D structure became available [49]. In the last few years, research has been concentrated on seeking TS inhibitors directed to the sialic acid-binding site, but success has not yet been achieved.

The strongest inhibitor found so far is 6-chloro-9,10-dihydro-4,5,7-trihydroxy-9,10-dioxo-2-anthracenecarboxylic acid [55]. One matter of concern is that, in general, TS inhibitor effects in cell cultures or animal models have not been demonstrated. Additionally, no inhibitor has been developed to prevent TS interactions through non-catalytic regions. Thus, future studies are needed to develop effective inhibitors against TS and consequently open new prospects for treatments against Chagas disease.

Antioxidant Metabolism

Trypanothione ($T(SH)_2$) has a central role in trypanosomatid antioxidant mechanisms. $T(SH)_2$, a low molecular weight dithiol, is synthesized by trypanothione synthetase (TS), an enzyme absent in the vertebrate host. In the intricate trypanothione-dependent network, $T(SH)_2$ is maintained in its reduced form by a NADPH dependent flavoenzyme, trypanothione reductase (TR). This system replaces the glutathione and glutathione reductase intracellular thiol-redox system present in the vertebrate host. However, TR shows enough structural differences from GR to be chosen as a good drug target for the development of a specific therapy. $T(SH)_2$ is able to transfer reducing equivalents to tryparedoxin, glutathione or dehydroascorbate, which transfer the reducing equivalents to peroxidases, leading to the reduction of peroxides [reviewed in 56].

Five distinct peroxidases have been identified in *T. cruzi*, with distinct substrate specificity and intracellular locations. Tryparedoxin peroxidases are located in the cytosol (TcCPx) and in the mitochondrion (TcMPx) with low homology (57%) between the two and are involved in the detoxification of H_2O_2 and small chain organic hydroperoxides [57] and peroxynitrite [58]. Ascorbate peroxidase (APx) also detoxifies H_2O_2 and is located in the endoplasmic reticulum [reviewed in 56]. Finally, glutathione peroxidase-I (cytosol and glycosome) and -II (endoplasmic reticulum) confer resistance against phospholipid and fatty acid hydroperoxides [59]. When compared to the antioxidant mechanism present in the vertebrate host, this system, centered at $T(SH)_2$, has unique features that justify the labeling part of this system as potential targets for the development of selective trypanosomatid drugs.

A complementary role in *T. cruzi*'s antioxidant system is fulfilled by superoxide dismutase (SOD), which catalyzes the conversion of O_2^- to H_2O_2. *T. cruzi* has four types of SOD that are common to all trypanosomatids. The limited ability of O_2^- to cross biological membranes is justified by the presence of SOD in different intracellular compartments. In *T. cruzi*, 4 isoforms of SOD were described [60], but only two, SODA (mitochondrion) and SODB (cytosolic), have been cloned and characterized.

Taken all together, the antioxidant defense system enables *T. cruzi* to address ROS and reactive nitrogen species (RNS) that are generated by the host immune system [reviewed in 61] and from its own metabolism. The capacity of *T. cruzi* to address the host oxidative response is directly correlated to the success of the invasion process and the establishment of disease [62]. Supporting this, proteins of the antioxidant system, TcCPx, TcMPx, TS, cytosolic tryparedoxin (TPNI) and SOD are upregulated during the metacyclogenesis process [62, reviewed in 61]. This increase in expression enables the parasite to address the highly oxidative environment of macrophages.

Additionally, a significant correlation between these highlighted proteins and virulence was found [62]. Interestingly, TcCPx, but not TcMPx, could be detected in the incubation medium of H_2O_2- treated trypomastigotes [63]. Moreover, TcCPx and TcMPx in tissue-culture derived trypomastigotes can be modulated via oxidative stress, showing different expression patterns, suggesting that each peroxiredoxin may play a distinct role in protecting the parasite against oxidative stress [63].

Taking into consideration the importance of the antioxidant system for parasite survival, research groups have developed inhibitors to act on this system. In terms of "drugability," tryparedoxin and tryparedoxin peroxidases are ruled out because they interact with each other and both proteins have to interact with more than one protein as described above [reviewed in 64]. "Drugability" can be applied to TR and a variety of TR inhibitors found. However, their efficacies were disappointing [reviewed in 64]. Some of them were aimed at *T. brucei* TR, and because TR from these species have a high similarity to *T. cruzi* TR, they may be used interchangeably for structure-based inhibitor design and high-throughput screening [65]. Some examples are quinolines [66] and diaryl sulfide-based inhibitors [67]. The most attractive target is TS, but no effective inhibitors have yet been found [reviewed in 64].

Taking all this into consideration, highly specific and very potent inhibitors for the enzymes of the antioxidant network are needed to inhibit one enzyme; a significant inhibition of *T. cruzi* viability would be observed. A good alternative could be the use of multi-target drugs against several enzymes of this pathway. Still, the role of the antioxidant enzymes in the virulence and survival of *T. cruzi* under different environmental conditions and their indication as pharmacological targets justifies further investigation of these enzymes.

Final Considerations

The biology of *T. cruzi* has been intensively studied, allowing for the translation of basic scientific knowledge into a number of selected targets for the development of an improved therapy. Herein, some candidates were depicted showing the strategy used by the parasite to overcome the absence of an enzyme, as in the case of sialidase, where the parasite scavenges sialic acid from the host and transfers them to its surface; in this way, the parasite avoids the immune response triggered by the host, to the presence of molecules with low homology when compared to those present in the vertebrate host and some unique proteins that participate in elaborate pathways, such as trypanothione and trypanothione reductase, which substitute the glutathione/glutathione reductase system present in the mammalian host. Unfortunately, despite the uniqueness of some molecules or the absence of important biosynthetic enzymes, very few effective inhibitors have been found, and only a small proportion of them have entered clinical trials. In light of the results obtained so far, Chagas disease still remains a challenge for the development of a more effective chemotherapy

References

[1]   Dumonteil E, Bottazzi ME, Zhan B, Heffernan MJ, Jones K, Valenzuela JG, Kamhawi S, Ortega J, Rosales SPL, Lee BY, Bacon KM, Fleischer B, Slingsby BT, Cravioto MB, Tapia-Conyer R, Hotez PJ. Accelerating the development of a therapeutic vaccine for human Chagas disease: rationale and prospects. *Expert Rev. Vaccines.* 2012; 11: 1043–55.

[2]   Barrett MP, Mottram JC, Coombs GH. Recent advances in identifying and validating drug targets in trypanosomes and leishmanias. *Trends in Microb.* 1999; 7(2): 82-8.

[3]   Vassena CV, Picollo MI, Zerba EN. Insecticide resistance in brazilian *Triatoma infestans* and Venezuelan *Rhodnius prolixus. Med. Vet. Entomol.* 2000; 14, 51–5.

[4]   Myler PJ. Searching the Tritryp genomes for drug targets. A*dv. Exp. Med. Biol.* 2008; 625: 133-40.

[5]   Pink R, Hudson A, Mouries MA. Opportunities and challenges in antiparasitic drug discovery. *Nat. ver. Drug discov.* 2005; 4 (9) 727-40.

[6]   El Sayed NM, Myler PJ, Bartholomeu DC, Nilsson D, Aggarwal G, Tran AN, Ghedin E, Worthey EA, Delcher AL, Blandin G, Westenberger SJ,

Caler E, Cerqueira GC, Branche C, Haas B, Anupama A, Arner E, Aslund L, Attipoe P, Bontempi E, Bringaud F, Burton P, Cadag E, Campbell DA, Carrington M, Crabtree J, Darban H, da Silveira JF, de Jong P, Edwards K, Englund PT, Fazelina G, Feldblyum T, Ferella M, Frasch AC, Gull K, Horn D, Hou L, Huang Y, Kindlund E, Klingbeil M,Kluge S, Koo H, Lacerda D, Levin MJ, Lorenzi H, Louie T, Machado CR, McCulloch R, McKenna A, Mizuno Y, Mottram JC, Nelson S, Ochaya S, Osoegawa K, PaiG, Parsons M, Pentony M, Pettersson U, Pop M, Ramirez JL, Rinta J, Robertson L, Salzberg SL, Sanchez DO, Seyler A, Sharma R, Shetty J, Simpson AJ, Sisk E,Tammi MT, Tarleton R, Teixeira S, Van Aken S, Vogt C, Ward PN, Wickstead B, Wortman J, White O, Fraser CM, Stuart KD, Andersson B. The genome sequence of Tryp*anosoma cruzi*, etiologic agent of Chagas disease. *Science.* 2005; 309(5733): 409-15.

[7]   Opperdoes FR, Michels PA. Enzymes of carbohydrate metabolism as potential drug targets. *Int. J. Parasitol.* 2001; 31(5-6): 482-90.

[8]   Igoillo-Esteve M, Maugeri D, Stern AL, Beluardi P, Cazzulo JJ. The pentose phosphate pathway in *Trypanosoma cruzi*: a potential target for the chemotherapy of Chagas disease. *An. Acad. Bras. Cienc.* 2007; 79(4): 649-63.

[9]   Verlinde CL, Hannaert V, Blonski C, Willson M, Périé JJ, Fothergill-Gilmore LA, Opperdoes FR, Gelb MH, Hol WG, Michels PA. Glycolysis as a target for the design of new anti-trypanosome drugs. *Drug Resist. Updat.* 2001; 4(1): 50-65.

[10]   Urbina JA, Docampo R. Specific chemotherapy of Chagas disease: controversies and advances. *Trends Parasitol.* 2003; 19(11): 495-501.

[11]   Lepesheva GI, Waterman MR. Sterol 14alpha-demethylase (CYP51) as a therapeutic target for human Trypanosomiasis and Leishmaniasis. *Curr. Top. Med. Chem.* 2011; 11(16): 2060–71.

[12]   Kavanagh KL, Guo K, Dunford JE, Wu X, Knapp S, Ebetino FH, Rogers MJ, Russell RG, Oppermann U. The molecular mechanism of nitrogen-containing bisphosphonates as antiosteoporosis drugs. *Proc. Natl. Acad. Sci. USA.* 2006; 103(20): 7829–34.

[13]   Cammerer SB, Jimenez C, Jones S, Gros L, Lorente SO, Rodrigues C, Rodrigues JC, Caldera A, Ruiz Perez LM, da Souza W, Kaiser M, Brun R, Urbina JA, Gonzalez Pacanowska D, Gilbert IH. Quinuclidine derivatives as potential antiparasitics. *Antimicrob. Agents Chemother.* 2007; 51(11): 4049–61.

[14] de Souza W, Rodrigues JC. Sterol Biosynthesis Pathway as target for anti-trypanosomatid drugs. *Interdiscip_Perspect Infect. Dis.* 2009; 2009: 642502.

[15] Zonios DI, Bennet JE. Update on azole antifungals. *Semin Respir Crit Care Med.* 2008; 29: 198–210.

[16] Zhivotovsky B, Orrenius S. Calcium and cell death mechanisms: A perspective from the cell death community. *Cell. Calcium* 2011; 50: 211-21.

[17] Benaim G, Garcia CRS. Targeting calcium homeostasis as the therapy of Chagas'disease and leishmaniasis − a review. *Trop. Biomed.* 2011; 28(3): 471-81.

[18] Bowles DJ, Voorheis H P (1982). Release of the surface coat from the plasma membrane of intact bloodstream forms of *Trypanosoma brucei* requires Ca^{2+}. *FEBS Letters.* 1982; 139: 17-21.

[19] D'Angelo MA, Montagna AE, Sanguineti S, Torres HN, Flawia MM. A novel calcium stimulated adenylyl cyclase from *Trypanosoma cruzi*, which interacts with the structural flagellar protein paraflagellar rod. *J. Biol. Chem.* 2002; 277: 35025-34.

[20] Tellez-Iñon MT, Ulloa RM, Torruela M, Torres HN. Calmodulin and Ca^{2+}-dependent cyclic AMP phosphodiesterase activity in *Trypanosoma cruzi. Mol. Biochem. Parasitol.* 1985; 17: 143-53.

[21] Stojdl DF, Clarke MW. (1996). *Trypanosoma brucei:* analysis of cytoplasmic Ca^{2+} during differentiation of bloodstream stages in vitro. *Exp. Parasitol.* 1996; 83: 134-46.

[22] Naderer T, Dandash O, McConville MJ. Calcineurin is required for *Leishmania major* stress response pathways and for virulence in the mammalian host *Mol. Microb.* 2011; 80(2): 471–80.

[23] Moreno SNJ, Vercesi AE, Docampo R. Cytosolic-free calcium elevation in *Trypanosoma cruzi* is required for cell invasion. *J. Exp. Med.* 1994; 180: 1535-40.

[24] Lu HG, Zhong L, Chang KP, Docampo R. Intracellular Ca^{2+} pool content and signaling and expression of a calcium pump are linked to virulence in *Leishmania mexicana amazonesis* amastigotes. *J._Biol. Chem.* 1997; 272(14): 9464-73.

[25] Sajid M, McKerrow JH. Cysteine proteases of parasitic organisms. *Mol. Biochem. Parasitol.* 2002; 120: 1–21.

[26] Caffrey CR, Scory S, Steverding D. Cysteine proteinases of Trypanosome parasites: novel targets for chemotherapy. *Curr. Drug Targets.* 2000; 1: 155-62.

[27] Huete-Perez JA, Engel JC, Brinen LS, Mottram JC, McKerrow JH. (1999) Protease trafficking in two primitive eukaryotes is mediated by a prodomain protein motif. *J. Biol Chem.* 1999; 274(23): 16249-56.

[28] Doyle PS, Zhou YM, Hsieh I, Greenbaum DC, McKerrow JH, Engel JC. The *Trypanosoma cruzi* protease cruzain mediates immune evasion. *PLoS Pathog.* 2011; 7(9): e1002139.

[29] Yong V, Schmitz V, Vannier-Santos MA, de Lima AP, Lalmanach G, Juliano L, Gauthier F, Scharfstein J. Altered expression of cruzipain and a cathepsin B-like target in a *Trypanosoma cruzi* cell line displaying resistance to synthetic inhibitors of cysteineproteinases. *Mol. Biochem. Parasitol.* 2000; 109: 47–59.

[30] Aoki MP, Cano RC, Pellegrini AV, Tanos T, Guinazu NL, Coso OA, Gea S. (2006) Different signaling pathways are involved in cardiomyocyte survival induced by a *Trypanosoma cruzi* glycoprotein. *Microbes Infect.* 2006; 8: 1723–31.

[31] Duschak VG, Ciaccio M, Nassert JR, Basombrio MA. Enzymatic activity, protein expression, and gene sequence of cruzipain in virulent and attenuated *Trypanosoma cruzi* strains. *J. Parasitol.* 2001; 87: 1016–22.

[32] Engel JC, Doyle PS, Hsieh I, McKerrow JH. Cysteine protease inhibitors cure an experimental *Trypanosoma cruzi* infection. *J. Exp. Med.* 1998; 188: 725–34.

[33] National Institute of Allergy and Infectious diseases (on line) Available from: http://www.niaid.nih.gov/about/organization/dmid/success/Pages/K777.aspx.

[34] Müller S, Coombs GH, Walter RD. Targeting polyamines of parasitic protozoa in chemotherapy. *Trends Parasitol.* 2001; 17(5):242-9.

[35] Barclay JJ, Morosi LG, Vanrell MC, Trejo EC, Romano PS, Carrillo C. *Trypanosoma cruzi* coexpressing ornithine decarboxylase and green fluorescence protein as a tool to study the role of polyamines in chagas disease pathology. *Enzyme Res.* 2011; 2011: 657460.

[36] González NS, Huber A, Algranati ID. Spermidine is essential for normal proliferation of trypanosomatid protozoa. *FEBS Lett.* 2001; 508(3): 323-6.

[37] Birkholtz LM, Williams M, Niemand J, Louw AI, Persson L, Heby O. Polyamine homoeostasis as a drug target in pathogenic protozoa: peculiarities and possibilities. *Biochem. J.* 2011; 438(2): 229-44.

[38] Castillo E, Dea-Ayuela MA, Bolás-Fernández F, Rangel M, González-Rosende ME. The kinetoplastid chemotherapy revisited: current drugs,

recent advances and future perspectives *Curr. Med. Chem.* 2010; 17: 4027-51.

[39] Yakubu, M. A., Majumder, S. and Kierszenbaum, F. (1993) Inhibition of S -adenosyl- 1 -methionine (AdoMet) decarboxylase by the decarboxylated AdoMet analog 5-([(Z)-4-amino-2-butenyl] methylamino)-5-deoxyadenosine (MDL73811) decreases the capacities of *Trypanosoma cruzi* to infect and multiply within a mammalian host cell. *J. Parasitol.* 1993; 79: 525–32.

[40] Szöör B. Trypanosomatid protein phosphatases. *Mol. Biochem. Parasitol,* 2010; 173: 53–63.

[41] Hunter T. Protein kinases and phosphatases: the yin and yang of protein phosphorylation and signaling. *Cell.* 1995; 80: 225–36.

[42] Huang H. Signal transduction in *Trypanosoma cruzi. Adv. Parasitol.* 2011; 75: 325–44.

[43] Brenchley R, Tariq H, McElhinney H, Szoor B, Huxley-Jones J, Stevens R, et al. The TriTryp phosphatome: analysis of the protein phosphatase catalytic domains. *BMC Genomics* 2007; 8: 434.

[44] Barford D, Flint AJ, Tonks NK. Crystal structure of human protein tyrosine phosphatase 1B, *Science.* 1994; 263: 1397–404.

[45] Gallo G, Ramos TC, Tavares F, Rocha AA, Machi E, Schenkman S, et al. Biochemical characterization of a protein tyrosine phosphatase from *Trypanosoma cruzi* involved in metacyclogenesis and cell invasion. *Biochem. Biophys. Res. Commun.* 2011; 408: 427–31.

[46] Lountos GT, Tropea JE, Waugh DS. Structure of the *Trypanosoma cruzi* protein tyrosine phosphatase TcPTP1, a potential therapeutic target for Chagas' disease. *Mol. Biochem. Parasitol.* 2013; 187: 1–8.

[47] Schenkman RP, Vandekerckhove F, Schenkman S. Mammalian cell sialic acid enhances invasion by *Trypanosoma cruzi. Infect. Immun.* 1993; 61: 898–902.

[48] Pereira-Chioccola VL, Acosta-Serrano A, Correia de Almeida I, Ferguson MA, Souto-Padron T, Rodrigues MM, Travassos LR, Schenkman S. Mucin-like molecules form a negatively charged coat that protects *Trypanosoma cruzi* trypomastigotes from killing by human antialpha-galactosyl antibodies. *J. Cell Sci.* 2000; 113: 1299–307.

[49] Buschiazzo A, Amaya MF, Cremona ML, Frasch AC, Alzari PM. The crystal structure and mode of action of trans-sialidase, a key enzyme in *Trypanosoma cruzi* pathogenesis. *Mol. Cell.* 2002; 10: 757–68.

[50] Garcia ES, Azambuja P. Development and interactions of *Trypanosoma cruzi* within the insect vector. *Parasitol. Today.* 1991; 7: 240–4.

[51] Rubin-de-Celis SS, Uemura H, Yoshida N, Schenkman S. (2006) Expression of trypomastigote trans-sialidase in metacyclic forms of *Trypanosoma cruzi* increases parasite escape from its parasitophorous vacuole. *Cell. Microbiol.* 2006; 8: 1888–98.

[52] Taylor, G. Sialidases: structures, biological significance and therapeutic potential. *Curr. Opin. Struct. Biol.* 1996; 6: 830–7.

[53] Giorgi ME, de Lederkremer RM. Trans-sialidase and mucins of *Trypanosoma cruzi*: an important interplay for the parasite. *Carbohydr. Res.* 2011; 346(12): 1389-93.

[54] Neres J, Bryce RA, Douglas KT. Rational drug design in parasitology: trans-sialidase as a case study for Chagas disease. *Drug Discov Today.* 2008; 13(3-4): 110-7.

[55] Arioka S, Sakagami M, Uematsu R, Yamaguchi H, Togame H, Takemoto H, Hinou H, Nishimura S. Potent inhibitor scaffold against *Trypanosoma cruzi* trans-sialidase. *Bioorg. Med. Chem.* 2010; 18: 1633–40.

[56] Irigoín F, Cibils L, Comini MA, Wilkinson SR, Flohé L, Radi R. Insights into the redox biology of *Trypanosoma cruzi*: Trypanothione metabolism and oxidant detoxification. *Free Radic. Biol. Med.* 2008; 45(6): 733-42.

[57] Wilkinson SR, Temperton NJ, Mondragon A, Kelly JM. Distinct mitochondrial and cytosolic enzymes mediate trypanothione-dependent peroxide metabolism in *Trypanosoma cruzi. J. Biol. Chem.* 2000; 275: 8220–25.

[58] Pineyro MD, Arcari T, Robello C, Radi R, Trujillo M. Tryparedoxin peroxidases from *Trypanosoma cruzi*: high efficiency in the catalytic elimination of hydrogen peroxide and peroxynitrite. *Arch. Biochem. Biophys.* 2011; 507: 287–95.

[59] Wilkinson SR, Kelly JM. The role of glutathione peroxidases in trypanosomatids. *Biol. Chem.* 2003; 384: 517–25.

[60] Dufernez F, Yernaux C, Gerbod D, Noël C, Chauvenet M, Wintjens R, Edgcomb VP, Capron M, Opperdoes FR, Viscogliosi E. The presence of four iron containing superoxide dismutase isozymes in trypanosomatidae:characterization, subcellular localization, and phylogenetic origin in *Trypanosoma brucei. Free Radic. Biol. Med.* 2006; 40(2): 210-25.

[61] Piacenza L, Alvarez, MN, Peluffo, G and Radi R. Fighting the oxidative assault: the *Trypanosoma cruzi* journey to infection. *Curr. Opin. Microbiol.* 2009; 12: 415-21.

[62] Piacenza L, Zago MP, Peluffo G, Alvarez MN, Basombrio MA, Radi R. Enzymes of the antioxidant network as novel determinaers of *Trypanosoma cruzi* virulence. *Int. J. Parasitol.* 2009; 39: 1455–64.

[63] Gadelha FR, Gonçalves CC, Mattos EC, Alves MJ, Piñeyro MD, Robello C, Peloso EF. Release of the cytosolic tryparedoxin peroxidase into the incubation medium and a different profile of cytosolic and mitochondrial peroxiredoxin expression in H_2O_2-treated *Trypanosoma cruzi* tissue culture-derived trypomastigotes. *Exp. Parasitol.* 2013; 133(3): 287-93.

[64] Flohé L. The trypanothione system and the opportunities it offers to create drugs for the neglected kinetoplast diseases *Biotechnology advances*. 2012; 30(1): 294-301.

[65] Jones DC, Ariza A, Chow WH, Oza SL, Fairlamb AH. Comparative structural, kinetic and inhibitor studies of *Trypanosoma brucei*

[66] trypanothione reductase with *T. cruzi*. *Mol Biochem Parasitol.* 2010; 169(1): 12-9.

[67] Spinks D, Shanks EJ, Cleghorn LA, McElroy S, Jones D, James D, Fairlamb AH, Frearson JA, Wyatt PG, Gilbert IH. Investigation of trypanothione reductase as a drug target in *Trypanosoma brucei*. *Chem. Med. Chem.* 2009; 4: 2060–69.

[68] Stump B, Eberle C, Kaiser M, Brun R, Krauth-Siegel RL, Diederich F. Diaryl sulfide-based inhibitors of trypanothione reductase: inhibition potency, revised binding mode and antiprotozoal activities. *Org. Biomol. Chem.* 2008; 6: 3935–47.

Index

Q

R

S